OXFORD SPECIALIST HANDBOOK OF

Old Age Psychiatry

Oxford Specialist Handbooks published and forthcoming

General Oxford Specialist Handbooks

Applied Medicine and Surgery in Dentistry 3e
Cardiopulmonary Transplantation and Mechanical Circulatory Support
Infection in the Immunocompromised Host
Perioperative Medicine 2e
Pharmaceutical Medicine 2e
Postoperative Complications 2e
Prison Medicine and Health
Retrieval Medicine

Oxford Specialist Handbooks in Anaesthesia

Anaesthesia for Emergency Care
Global Anaesthesia
Neuroanaesthesia and Neurocritical Care
Obstetric Anaesthesia 2e
Paediatric Anaesthesia 2e
Regional Anaesthesia, Stimulation, and Ultrasound Techniques
Thoracic Anaesthesia
Vascular Anaesthesia

Oxford Specialist Handbooks in Cardiology

Adult Congenital Heart Disease 2e
Cardiac Catheterization and Coronary Intervention 2e
Cardiovascular Computed Tomography 2e
Cardiovascular Imaging
Cardiovascular Magnetic Resonance
Echocardiography 3e
Fetal Cardiology 2e
Heart Disease in Pregnancy
Heart Failure, 3e
Inherited Cardiac Disease 2e
Nuclear Cardiology 2e
Pacemakers and ICDs 2e
Paediatric Cardiology
Pulmonary Hypertension
Valvular Heart Disease

Oxford Specialist Handbooks in End of Life Care

End of Life Care in Dementia
End of Life Care in Heart Failure
End of Life Care in Kidney Disease
End of Life Care in Respiratory Disease

Oxford Specialist Handbooks in Neurology

Clinical Neurophysiology
Neurointervention
Parkinson's Disease and Other Movement Disorders 2e
Stroke Medicine, 3e

Oxford Specialist Handbooks in Obstetrics and Gynaecology

Obstetric Medicine
Urogynaecology

Oxford Specialist Handbooks in Oncology

Myeloproliferative Neoplasms
Practical Management of Complex Cancer Pain 2e
Radiotherapy Planning

Oxford Specialist Handbooks in Paediatrics

Manual of Childhood Infections 4e
Neurodisability and Community Child Health 2e
Paediatric Dermatology 2e
Paediatric Endocrinology and Diabetes 2e
Paediatric Gastroenterology, Hepatology, and Nutrition 2e
Paediatric Haematology and Oncology 2e
Paediatric Intensive Care
Paediatric Nephrology 3e
Paediatric Neurology 4e
Paediatric Palliative Medicine 2e
Paediatric Respiratory Medicine 2e
Paediatric Rheumatology 2e

Oxford Specialist Handbooks in Psychiatry

Eating Disorders
Forensic Psychiatry 2e
Medical Psychotherapy
Old Age Psychiatry 2e

Oxford Specialist Handbooks in Radiology

Head and Neck Imaging
Interventional Radiology
Musculoskeletal Imaging
Thoracic Imaging

Oxford Specialist Handbooks in Surgery

Burns
Cardiothoracic Surgery 2e
Colorectal Surgery 2e
Current Surgical Guidelines 2e
Gastric and Oesophageal Surgery
Hand Surgery 2e
Oral and Maxillofacial Surgery 3e
Otolaryngology and Head and Neck Surgery
Paediatric Surgery 2e
Plastic and Reconstructive Surgery 2e
Urological Surgery 2e
Vascular Surgery 2e

Oxford Specialist Handbook of

Old Age Psychiatry

SECOND EDITION

Daniel Casey
Specialty Registrar in Old Age Psychiatry,
Oxford Health and Berkshire NHS, UK

Bart Sheehan
Consultant in Psychological Medicine,
John Radcliffe Hospital, Oxford, UK

OXFORD
UNIVERSITY PRESS

OXFORD
UNIVERSITY PRESS

Great Clarendon Street, Oxford, OX2 6DP,
United Kingdom

Oxford University Press is a department of the University of Oxford. It furthers the University's objective of excellence in research, scholarship, and education by publishing worldwide. Oxford is a registered trade mark of Oxford University Press in the UK and in certain other countries.

First Edition published in 2009
Second Edition published in 2026

Published in the United States of America by Oxford University Press
198 Madison Avenue, New York, NY 10016, United States of America.

British Library Cataloguing in Publication Data
Data available

Library of Congress Control Number: 2026933571

ISBN 978–0–19–888928–1

DOI: 10.1093/med/9780198889281.001.0001

Printed in India by
Replika Press Pvt. Ltd.

Preface

The world is ageing in a wave which is spreading at different rates over different continents and countries. There is increasing focus on the universal challenges this brings, in particular increased discussion of how a shrinking working age population can support an expanding population of retired, ageing, and increasingly frail older people. Advances in human longevity mean increased incidence of the great diseases of older age. Some psychiatric disorders like depressive disorders, chronic schizophrenia, and anxiety disorders are found just as commonly among older people as in the young but need a different approach as people age. Some, like dementia and delirium, become much more likely with advancing age. Achievements in extending life are not yet matched by prevention of disorders and no matter what is done, all societies will need to grapple with huge numbers of older people with these disorders. Most of that challenge will fall to family carers, to paid informal carers, or to healthcare professionals not specializing in psychiatry. Most people encountering healthcare with these disorders will be in care homes, primary care offices, or general hospitals. This can be seen as an opportunity. Actions can be taken in prevention, recognition, referral, and management which can all make a difference and need not be the province of the specialist. The task of old age psychiatry is probably to spread key messages among non-specialist colleagues. This handbook is aimed at helping those needing to make clinical decisions while knowing that their decisions make sense in the context of a changing world of demographics, science, and societal pressure. Might this person with no memory loss already have dementia? Is referral worth it now? If I can't refer them, what could I do? What does this episode of acute confusion mean for their future? If antidepressants make no difference to their mood, can anything be done? These can all seem daunting questions, but the answers are getting better and something wise can be done now. This book can only succeed if it helps the reader address their particular question quickly and simply.

Daniel Casey
Bart Sheehan

Preface

Contents

Detailed contents

Abbreviations

5-HT	5-hydroxytryptamine (serotonin)
ABRA	amyloid beta-related angiitis
ACE-III-R	Addenbrooke's Cognitive Examination III-revised
AChEI	acetylcholinesterase inhibitor
ACID	antidepressant-associated chronic irritable dysphoria
AD	Alzheimer's disease
AD	antidepressant
ADAS	Alzheimer's Disease Assessment Scale
ADLs	activities of daily living
AE	adverse event
AIMS	Abnormal Involuntary Movement Scale
aMCI	amnestic MCI
aMRI	amnestic MRI
AMT	Abbreviated Mental Test
APOE	apolipoprotein E
APP	amyloid precursor protein
ARIAs	amyloid-related imaging abnormalities
BADLS	Bristol Activities of Daily Living Scale
BD	*bis die* (twice daily)
BPRS	Brief Psychiatric Rating Scale
BEHAVE-AD	Behavioural Pathology in Alzheimer's Disease rating scale
BP	bipolar
BPSD	behavioural and psychological symptoms of dementia
BOLD	blood oxygen level dependent
bvAD	behavioural variant AD
CAA	cerebral amyloid angiopathy
CAM	Confusion Assessment Method
CAMCOG	Cambridge Cognitive Examination
CAM-S	Confusion Assessment Method—Severity
CBD	corticobasal degeneration
CBS	corticobasal syndrome
CBS-AD	corticobasal syndrome AD
CBT	cognitive behavioural therapy
CCAS	cerebellar cognitive affective syndrome
CDR	Clinical Dementia Rating
CERAD	Consortium to Establish a Registry for Alzheimer's Disease
CES-D	Centre for Epidemiological Studies—Depression Scale
CGI-C	Clinical Global Impression scores of Change
CGI-S	Clinical Global Impression scores of Severity
CMAI	Cohen–Mansfield Agitation Inventory
CNS	central nervous system
CPAP	continuous positive air pressure
CPN	community psychiatric nurse
CRP	C-reactive protein
CSF	cerebrospinal fluid
CSTC	cortico-striato-thalamo-cortical
CT	computed tomography
CU	cognitively unimpaired
CVA	cerebrovascular accident
CVD	cardiovascular disease
DA	dopamine
DBS	dried blood spot
DBS	deep brain stimulation
DED	depression executive dysfunction
dexAD	dysexecutive AD
DLB	dementia with Lewy bodies
DLPFC	dorsolateral prefrontal cortex
DMN	default mode network
DoLs	Deprivation of Liberty safeguards
DORAs	dual orexin receptor antagonists
DPIVC	difficult peripheral intravenous cannulation
DSM	Diagnostic and Statistical Manual
DTI	diffusion tensor imaging
DWML	deep white matter lesion
ECT	electroconvulsive therapy
EEG	electroencephalogram
EOBP	early-onset bipolar
EOS	early-onset schizophrenia
EPA	Enduring Power of Attorney

EPS	extrapyramidal symptoms
ESR	erythrocyte sedimentation rate
FAB	Frontal Assessment Battery
FBI	Frontal Behavioural Inventory
FDA	US Food and Drug Administration
FDG-PET	fluorodeoxyglucose-PET
FEP	fist–edge–palm
FGA	first-generation antipsychotic
FLAIR	fluid attenuated inversion recovery
fMRI	functional MRI
FTD	fronto-temporal dementia
FTLD	frontotemporal lobar degeneration
GABA	gamma-aminobutyric acid
GAD	generalized anxiety disorder
GAGE-BD	Global Aging & Geriatric Experiments in Bipolar Disorder
GCA	global cortical atrophy
GDS	Geriatric Depression Scale
GFAP	glial fibrillary acidic protein
GP	General Practitioner
H&E	haematoxylin and eosin
HD	hoarding disorder
HD	Huntington's disease
HDRS	Hamilton Depression Rating Scale
HMPAO	hexamethylpropyleneamine oxime
ICD	impulse control disorder
ICD	International Classification of Diseases
ICU	intensive care unit
IDS	Inventory of Depressive Symptomatology
IM	intramuscular
IMCA	Independent mental capacity advocate
IPSRT	interpersonal and social rhythm therapy
IQCODE	Informant Questionnaire on Cognitive Decline in the Elderly
IV	intravenous
IWG	International Working Group
LATE	limbic-predominant age-related TDP-43 encephalopathy
LFT	liver function test
LLD	late-life depression
LOBP	late-onset bipolar
LOS	late-onset schizophrenia
LP	lumbar puncture
LPA	Lasting Power of Attorney
LPS	Liberty Protection safeguards
lvPPA	logopenic variant of primary progressive aphasia
MADRS	Montgomery and Asberg Depression Rating Scale
MAOI	monoamine oxidase inhibitors
MBI-C	Mild Behavioural Impairment Checklist
MCI	mild cognitive impairment
MDAS	Memorial Delirium Assessment Scale
MDD	major depressive disorder
MIBG	meta-iodobenzylguanidine
MMSE	Mini Mental State Examination
MoCA	Montreal Cognitive Assessment
MRI	magnetic resonance imaging
MSA	multiple system atrophy
MSU	mid-stream specimen of urine
MT	motor threshold
MTA	medial temporal lobe atrophy
naMCI	non-amnestic MCI
NBM	nucleus basalis of Meynert
NBRS	Neurobehavioral Rating Scale
NfL	neurofilament light chain
NFTs	neurofibrillary tangles
NIA-AA	National Institute on Aging and Alzheimer's Association
NIBS	non-invasive brain stimulation
NICE	National Institute for Health and Care Excellence
NIH	National Institute of Health
NMDA	N-methyl-D-aspartate
NPI	Neuropsychiatric Inventory
NPI-Q	Neuropsychiatric Inventory Questionnaire
NSAID	non-steroidal anti-inflammatory drug
OABP	older age bipolar disorder
OCD	obsessive–compulsive disorder
ON	once at night (*omni nocte*)
OPTIMUM	Optimizing Outcomes of Treatment-Resistant Depression in Older Adults
PAMs	positive allosteric modulators
PART	primary age-related tauopathy
PBA	pseudobulbar affect
PC	presenting complaint
PCA	posterior cortical atrophy

PD	Parkinson's disease
PDD	Parkinson's disease dementia
PEG	percutaneous endoscopic gastrostomy
PET	positron emission tomography
PHQ	Patient Health Questionnaire
PPA	primary progressive aphasia
PRN	as required (*pro re nata*)
PSD	post-stroke dementia
PSEN	presenilin
PSP	progressive supranuclear palsy
PST	problem-solving therapy
PTSD	post-traumatic stress disorder
QIDS	Quick Inventory of Depressive Symptomatology
Qmci	Quick mild cognitive impairment screen
RAADs	rapid acting antidepressants
RAVLT-DR	Rey Auditory Verbal Learning Test
RBD	rapid eye movement sleep behaviour disorder
RCT	randomized controlled trial
REM	rapid eye movement
RMS	Rapid Mood Screener
RPLS	reversible posterior leukoencephalopathy syndrome
rTMS	repetitive transcranial magnetic stimulation
SAPS–H+D	Scale for the Assessment of Positive Symptoms—Hallucinations and Delusions
SASP	senescence-associated secretory phenotype
SCD	subjective cognitive decline
SGA	second-generation antipsychotics
SIADH	syndrome of inappropriate antidiuretic hormone secretion
SNRIs	serotonin and norepinephrine reuptake inhibitors
SPECT	single-photon emission computed tomography
SSRIs	selective serotonin reuptake inhibitors
SWS	slow wave sleep
TBI	traumatic brain injury
TCA	tricyclic antidepressants
TD	tardive dyskinesia
TEMPS	Temperament Scale of Memphis, Pisa, Paris and San Diego
TFT	thyroid function test
TGA	Transient Global Amnesia
THA	tetrahydroaminoacridine
TIA	transient ischaemic attack
TMS	transcranial magnetic stimulation
TPS	transcranial pulse stimulation
TRD	treatment-resistant depression
TS	total score
U&E	urea and electrolytes
UTI	urinary tract infection
VaD	vascular dementia
VaDeP	vascular depression
VCI	vascular cognitive impairment
VH	visual hallucinations
VICCCS	Vascular Impairment of Cognition Classification Consensus Study
VLOSLP	very-late-onset schizophrenia-like psychosis
VMAT	vesicular monoamine transporter
VNS	vagal nerve stimulation
WMH	white matter hyperintensities
XR	extended release
YMRS	Young Mania Rating Scale
YOD	young-onset dementia

Chapter 1

Introduction

History of a specialty

Old age psychiatry developed as a specialty, especially in the UK, from the 1980s. The concept of old age psychiatry would have seemed odd until at least the 1960s, when a wider appreciation arose that older people did not just suffer from an amorphous entity called senility but rather had distinct illnesses with different aetiologies, outcomes, and even treatments. The key observations were of asylum populations where it could be shown that some had dementia (with a relentlessly progressive course of deterioration), some had schizophrenia (with a negative defect state in some cases but in others distinct phases of acute illness followed by recovery), and depression (in which some older people would deteriorate to a dangerous degree due to catatonia, starvation, or dehydration, but in many or most cases there would be recovery due to time or treatment, and no clear defect state or cognitive impairment). Realization of this basic epidemiology coincided with the development of modern treatments—from the 1950s on when antidepressants and antipsychotics were introduced, to the refinement of previously primitive treatment with electroconvulsive therapy (ECT). Ageing populations, and political will, led to increased interest in, and funding of, old age psychiatry teams, and particular impetus came from dawning realization that there was a cholinergic deficit in Alzheimer's disease (AD) and rational treatment in the form of cholinesterase inhibitors became available in the 1990s. Around this time structural imaging in the form of computed tomography (CT) and magnetic resonance imaging (MRI) became widely available and interest in specificity of diagnoses rose, leading to the establishment of specialist memory services in many countries.

There has been a frustrating delay in new disease modifying treatments coming on line since, but the US licensing of the amyloid lowering agents aducanumab (in 2021), lecanemab (in 2023) and donanemab (in 2024) has generated new impetus. Despite ageing populations, there has been an increased focus on age-independent services in mental health, especially in the UK. In practice, this rarely makes sense once the importance of the major organic syndromes of dementia and delirium is understood.

As knowledge of delirium and dementia develops, and new health technologies such as cerebrospinal fluid (CSF) protein assays, specialist imaging, and disease-modifying treatments come onstream, the battle may be to keep the specialty within the bounds of psychiatry rather than neurology. This handbook focuses on the skills and knowledge needed to be effective now and in the future at a time when even the monolith which is dementia at last appears capable of being chipped away by treatment.

Overview of mental disorder among older people in different settings

Perspectives on which older people have a mental disorder have changed greatly with time. In the 1950s, mental illness among older people would have conjured up images of long-stay wards with dormitory arrangements in the old asylums. Increased interest in epidemiological research, in part driven by an ageing population, has delineated the prevalence of psychiatric disorders in different settings. Old age psychiatrists and community mental health teams tend to see equal numbers of new cases of dementia and functional psychiatric illness. In-patient bed provision is typically about equally occupied by dementia and functional cases. Dementia, by its progressive nature, tends to accrete and the caseloads of community teams could typically have far more long-term patients with dementia. Provision of long-stay care for people with dementia in the UK initially moved from hospital care to local authority care homes but now is almost exclusively provided in privately run residential and nursing homes. Dementia is usual in residents of residential and nursing homes, even those in non-specialist elderly frail care homes. About 200 000 to 250 000 people with dementia now live in care homes in the UK. Depression is common in this setting, with prevalence estimates between 20% and 40%, but this may resolve, especially with appropriate treatment.

In primary care, where most care is delivered, the situation is different. Over 90% of older people in the UK consult with their GP each year, allowing unique case-finding opportunities. An average GP will have about 35 cases of dementia on their caseload at any time (not all identified), roughly similar to the numbers with declared rheumatoid arthritis or epilepsy. Five to ten new cases of possible or probable dementia may be identified and referred by a GP in a year.

Many cases of psychiatric illness never declare to services. Table 1.1 gives the approximate known prevalence of psychiatric disorders in various settings. It can be assumed that these figures are similar across developed countries. European studies of the prevalence of depression and dementia in the community confirm this. In the developing world, the population is ageing much more rapidly than has ever been seen in the West. Early epidemiological work shows that the prevalence of dementia, and the social consequences of it, are similar among older people in developing countries. Services are rudimentary or non-existent in such countries, leaving people with dementia even more dependent on their families than in developed countries.

Table 1.1 Prevalence of common psychiatric disorders among older people by setting

	Dementia	Depression	Delirium
Emergency general hospital admissions	20–40%	12–20%	15%
Residential/nursing homes	50–60%	20–40%	5%
Primary care older attendees	5–10%	10–20%	unknown
Community	5–7%	10–15%	unknown

Tips on assessing an older person with psychiatric disorder: 1

General

Take time

Assessment of older people with psychiatric disorder may take some time[1]. Collateral history will usually be required, while deafness or frailty will prolong assessments. Patients may well have multiple medical, social, and psychiatric problems, increasing assessment time. Patience and planning of assessment times will be needed.

Collateral history

In any psychiatric assessment, a collateral history is desirable. Among older people with cognitive impairment it is essential. In practice, most older people are happy to allow this. A breach of confidentiality is justified if information is required to help maintain the person's safety. Family members, social and health-care staff, or care home staff are invaluable sources of information. Key questions may include: 'How long has she been forgetful?' 'Has she been repeating herself more?' 'Has she locked herself out?' 'Has she left the gas on?' 'Has she been more irritable or resistant?' Attention may need to be paid to inclusion of the older person in the assessment, rather than just interviewing the informant.

Reduce distractions

Noisy hospital wards are among the worst places to take a history and assess a patient with dementia. Reducing outside noise, minimizing sensory impairments (putting in teeth/hearing aids/spectacles), going to a quiet room, switching off electronic devices will all be helpful.

Repetition

For those who are frail, deaf, or cognitively impaired, repetition may be needed. This may help to maintain dignity or establish facts. Sometimes it is strategic; for example, in deciding on capacity issues: an older person may forget the detail of what was discussed but may on two separate occasions show clear evidence of capacity so the decision is valid even if forgotten in between

Mental state examination

The structure of mental state examination among older people is the same as with younger people. The emphases within each component are different and are outlined below.

Appearance and behaviour

- Are there signs of recent weight loss? Is there resting tremor? Is there agitation (more common in depression in old age)? Does the person show distractibility/poor attention span (common in dementia)? Do they defer to a carer (common in cognitive impairment)?

Speech

- Are they dysarthric (common in Parkinson's disease, motor neuron disease, after stroke, but also in the edentulous)? Are they dysphasic (very common after stroke or as part of a wider picture of impairment in dementia)? Are they repetitive (common in any dementia)?

Affect

- Are they markedly low (severe, psychotic depression is more common in old age and often accompanied by agitation and/or psychomotor retardation)?

Thoughts

- Is there insight into the extent of cognitive impairment and social care needed (frequently deficient in dementia)? Does the person have particular mood congruent delusions (very common in old age depression—especially nihilistic and hypochondriacal delusions)?

Perceptions

- Are there visual hallucinations (characteristic of dementia with Lewy Bodies (DLB))? Do they appear distracted by illusions/hallucinations (common in delirium)?

Cognition

- The ability to make a meaningful assessment of cognitive state is essential when assessing older people. Sometimes this is translated as ability to use the Montreal Cognitive Assessment (MoCA) or MMSE, but other instruments may be more appropriate. For example, the Abbreviated Mental Test score has good sensitivity to change and is often used to demonstrate fluctuating impairment in delirious patients on general hospital wards. The Memory Alteration Test has a high sensitivity for mild cognitive impairment (MCI). Scales such as the Addenbrooke's Cognitive Examination III-revised (ACE-III-R) and the Cambridge Cognitive Examination (CAMCOG) give a more detailed assessment of cognitive impairment, allowing domains of memory, orientation, speech, abstract thinking, attention/calculation, and visuospatial skills to be mapped. These scales can be useful when patients have more subtle deficits or have a high level of educational attainment. It is sometimes mistakenly thought that a poor score on a cognitive test means a diagnosis of dementia—it does not. At best these instruments are used as screening instruments for significant impairment and as a baseline which may be useful in plotting progress, for example in borderline cases or people on anti-dementia drugs.

Reference

1. Bowker LK, Price JD, Smith SC, et al. *Clinical assessment of older people. In: Oxford Handbook of Geriatric Medicine*. Oxford, Oxford University Press, 2006; 70–73.

Tips on assessing an older person with psychiatric disorder: 2, Physical examination

Some consideration of the patient's physical state should always be made. The prevalence of comorbid physical illness is very high among older psychiatric patients, and physical disorder may be directly relevant to the assessment. For example, if older people with cognitive impairment are hypertensive, have atrial fibrillation, and show localized neurological signs like dysphasia or hemiplegia, the likelihood of vascular dementia is higher. If a patient with dementia reports hallucinations and shows cogwheel rigidity, then DLB is more likely. If an older person with severe depression shows evidence of malnutrition and dehydration then urgent admission for ECT may be required.

The list below should be tailored to the individual case being assessed; not every psychiatric assessment needs all these examinations. The ability to do a comprehensive psychiatric assessment should be accompanied by the skill to do each of these examinations when needed.

System

General examination

- Hygiene: Any signs of recent weight loss? Alert? Do they look generally ill?

Systemic disease

- Any jaundice (examine sclerae). Any anaemia? Lymph glands enlarged? Any thyroid signs?

Skin/nails

- Are there any bruises (sign of falls/abuse)? Is skin turgor normal (may be dehydrated)? Any pressure sores (especially bed-bound people)?

Cardiovascular

- Check blood pressure. Is there any postural drop (consider checking this if the patient has been falling/dizzy)? Check pulse. Is there atrial fibrillation? Is the pulse weak and thready (if dehydrated)?

Respiratory

- Is the patient cyanosed? Is the respiratory rate increased (below 16/min is normal)? Are there any clear signs of infection, e.g. localized dullness/crepitations?

Abdomen

- Is there any organomegaly? Is there evidence of faecal loading? A rectal examination is essential if the person is constipated.

Central nervous system

- Is there any obvious sign of visual loss, especially visual field loss? Is downward gaze grossly impaired (found in some disorders causing parkinsonism)? Alcohol-dependent patients with Wernicke's encephalopathy may show grossly impaired eye movements.

- In the limbs, is there any clear hemiplegia? Check for reduced power, abnormal reflexes, and change in tone in limbs on either side. Is there cogwheel rigidity? Are gait and balance normal (gait ataxia is characteristic of normal pressure hydrocephalus)?

Musculo-skeletal

- Are any joints red/hot/swollen/painful? Is there clear deformity, e.g. ulnar deviation in fingers in rheumatoid arthritis. What restrictions in function do joint problems cause?

Demographics of ageing

The last century witnessed an unprecedented increase in the average human lifespan and population ageing has been described as a key 'mega trend' affecting the global population. The estimated total world population of older people was about 200 million in 1950 and is expected to rise to 1.5 billion by 2050. Currently, about 9% of the world's population comprises those aged 65 years or above, and this is expected to rise to 16% by 2050. The number of those aged 80 or over is expected to triple by 2050, reaching 426 million. There is wide variation across the world in the proportions of older people. Life expectancy from age 65 is expected to increase from 17 years in 2020 to 19 by 2040–2050.

The developing world

The developing world has a bigger proportion of children in the population (nearly 50% in some countries). The largest absolute increase in older persons is expected in South-East Asia, whereas the most rapid increase is expected in Western, Northern, and Sub-Saharan Africa (226% change between 2019 and 2050).

North America and Europe

The number of persons aged 65 or over is currently 200 million, and this is expected to increase by 48% to 296.2 million by 2050.

United Kingdom

In the UK over the last 35 years, the population aged over 65 grew by 31%, from 7.4 million to 9.7 million, whilst the population aged under 16 declined by 19%, from 14.2 million to 11.5 million. The proportion of people aged over 65 is projected to increase from 18.5% in 2019 to 25.3% by 2050.

Australia and New Zealand

By 2050, it is estimated that the number of persons aged 65 is expected to increase by 84% from 4.8 million to 8.8 million.

The ageing world

The reasons for this explosion in the older population in the world in general, and in the developed world in particular are many, and are not just a result of increasing life expectancy. Other factors including the declining fertility rate, declining child mortality, education, and economic development play a big part. The ageing population of the world presents major challenges for society and for health services. Health services will have to adapt to new demands of an ageing population as well as to associated costs.

Mental health in an ageing world

Mental health issues are extremely important, as mental disorders, notably dementia and depression, are common in old age. Mental ill-health can profoundly affect the quality of a person's old age and has a significant impact upon the use of health and social services.

Challenges in the developed world

Even in a developed country like the UK, with established mental health services for older people, repeated reports have shown that the mental health issues of older people remain poorly understood, highly stigmatized, and are not given the priority necessary in policy, practice, and research—despite official reports since at least 2000 highlighting discrimination and calling for action.

Two-thirds of older people with depression never even discuss it with their general practitioner or family doctor, and of the third that do discuss it, only less than half are diagnosed and treated. This means that of those with depression only approximately 15%, or one in seven, are diagnosed and receive any kind of treatment. Even when they are diagnosed, older people are less likely to be offered treatment, and depression is sometimes still regarded as an inherent symptom of growing older. With the rising numbers of older people there will be an estimated 3.5 million older people with symptoms of depression by 2050.

In the UK there are currently almost 1 million people with dementia, and this will rise to 1.7 million by 2050. Dementia affects one in five over 80, one in 14 aged over 65, and one in 79 of the UK population. The overall cost of dementia is £25 billion a year to the UK economy, and this will double by 2050. The current cost of dementia to the global economy is US $817 billion annually.

Challenges in the developing world

In the developing world an ageing of the population which is unprecedented in human history is now occurring. This is certain to place huge demands on social structures which will have to cope with increasing numbers of frail and unwell older people. In particular, assumptions that families will look after older relatives may be untenable. There is already evidence that mental health issues are of low priority in poorer countries with small health and social care budgets which are allocated across competing demands. Unrecognized and untreated mental illness may become a fate for many of those growing older in the developing world.

Epidemiology of mental disorders in old age

The epidemiology of mental disorders in old age is a rapidly evolving area. Most epidemiological research in this area has been conducted in Europe and North America. An overview of the prevalence of common mental disorders in old age will be given in this chapter.

Dementia

The prevalence of dementia increases with age. Most studies have shown a prevalence of 3% in the 70–75 year age group which increases exponentially to 20–25% in those aged 85+. The prevalence of AD differs across countries, with some studies suggesting a slightly higher prevalence of AD in older women than men, and a higher prevalence of vascular dementia in men.

Depression

Depression is common in old age and is considered the most treatable/reversible mental health disorder in old age. However, large survey data suggests a prevalence rate of depression of approximately 5% in those aged 60 or over, in comparison to 9.8% of those aged 40–60 and 7.4% for the 18–40 group. A systematic analysis of depression in latest life (75+) suggests a pooled prevalence of 7%.

There is, however, a general consensus that a number of methodological difficulties might have resulted in an underestimation of depression problems in epidemiological studies. The main confounders include exclusion of institutionalized individuals from sampling, diagnosis of dementia, and poor recognition of atypical depression when using the Diagnostic and Statistical Manual of Mental; Disorders (DSM) or International Classification of Diseases (ICD) criteria.

Anxiety disorders

There is a paucity of epidemiological research on other psychiatric disorders including anxiety, substance misuse, psychosis, and somatoform disorders in old age. Although these conditions are common in adult age groups, decreasing rates of anxiety disorders and substance misuse have been reported in older age. One survey suggested an overall prevalence of anxiety disorders of 17.2% (agoraphobia (4.9%), panic disorder (3.8%), animal phobia (3.5%), general anxiety disorder (3.1%), post-traumatic stress disorder (1.4%), social phobia (1.3%), and obsessive-compulsive disorder (0.8%)).

A number of methodological difficulties might account for decreasing rates of anxiety in older people. First, the current diagnostic assessment methods focusing on somatic symptoms of anxiety may not adequately differentiate between anxiety and symptoms of medical illness that are more common in the elderly. Secondly the assessment instruments are likely to miss comorbidity with other psychiatric disorders.

Drug abuse

Alcohol and drug abuse are consistently found to be less common among older people. This may be partly explained by premature deaths among substance abusers, by cohort effects (people in their 20s in the 1950s in the UK drank under half the amount of alcohol of their modern equivalents), and personal/societal distaste for substance use in older age.

Psychosis

Psychotic syndromes in later life appear to increase with age if a broader definition is used, but there is a paucity of epidemiological research on specific syndromes such as late-onset schizophrenia and delusional disorders. Psychotic symptoms in other disorders like depression and dementia are much more frequent than true paranoid illness in late life. It is also clear that the devastating effects of schizophrenia among younger people are rarely found among older people newly developing the condition. With an ageing population and no effective cure for dementia syndromes, psychosis in the context of behavioural and psychological symptoms of dementia (BPSD) is expected to increase significantly over the coming decades.

Normal ageing

There is no satisfactory definition of the normal ageing process. It can be defined as a cumulative process of adverse changes in physiological, psychological, and social functions that characterize average older people.

Normal ageing as a social concept refers to an accepted range of variation in health, appearance, and performance of adults at different stages of their lives. It is also a scientific concept referring to research findings in gerontology that can be useful in identifying variations from the normal ageing pattern. It is, however, always difficult to make a distinction between normal and pathological ageing.

Biological theories of ageing

According to biological theories the ageing process can be divided into primary and secondary ageing. *Primary ageing* refers to those declines in function that are genetically controlled and is the focus of 'program theories' whereas 'damage theories' focus on *secondary ageing*, which consists of random changes resulting from acquired disease and trauma. These theories suggest that if the hostile events related to secondary ageing could be prevented, life would be extended, but because of primary ageing decline and death are inevitable. There are several, interlinked 'pillars' or hallmarks of ageing which include: progenitor cell dysfunction, genomic and epigenetic changes, cellular senescence, mitochondrial dysfunction, and chronic inflammation.

Deliberate biological programming

Studies on the ageing processes of human cells have shown that mitotic cells can divide a finite number of times (Hayflick limit) and then die. Individual cells have a memory for the number of duplications, which is probably encoded in the genetic material. In other words, there exists a system of programmed cell death, thus making survival beyond a certain time limit impossible.

The ageing clock

This theory is based on the observation of biological clocks in both humans and animals. It suggests that ageing is a process that converts fit adults into frail adults with a progressively increased risk of illness, injury, and death. It refutes the concept of an absolute genetic control on the lifespan of an individual and suggests that living in favourable environments with positive living habits is the biggest influence on lifespan.

Accumulation theories

Other theories suggest that an accumulation of harmful substances such as free radicals and lipofuscin (an insoluble pigmented compound derived from incomplete degradation of normal cellular materials) with time result in an ageing process, eventually leading to death.

Cellular senescence

Senescent cells are in a state of cell cycle arrest, and can develop a senescence-associated secretory phenotype (SASP) which is harmful to the organism. The 'threshold theory of senescent cell accumulation' posits that accumulation over a certain point leads to a positive feedback loop of SASP induced senescence of non-senescent cells. One theory suggests that senolytic drugs targeting these senescent cells, which themselves resist apoptosis, can reverse this process.

Psychological theories of ageing

These can be broadly divided into cognitive and personality theories.

Cognitive theories

The cognitive theory is based on studies of cognitive changes associated with age. In general, adults with higher intelligence and education tend to show minimum decline in their performances with increasing age, while a significant decline is observed in adults with lower intelligence and education. Older adults in general tend to perform less well in new and novel situations. The decline in cognitive skills is neither inevitable nor universal and some skills may improve or may be acquired with age.

Whereas many might assume that old age might be associated with unhappiness, in fact there is evidence from different geographical populations that happiness follows a curved trajectory, with a nadir around age 49, and levels of happiness increasing with age thereafter. One hypothesis is that this is because, first, the developmental challenges of adult life have been completed and secondly, due to a cognitive process whereby the gap between unrealistic life expectations and reality gradually narrows until around mid-life, which then reverses such that reality is better than expected with each year.

Personality theories

CG Jung's psychological theory of ageing can be surmised as 'a human being would certainly not grow to be seventy or eighty years old if this longevity had no meaning for the species'. Erikson's famous eight-stage theory of ego development suggested that the elderly person might either find ego integrity through satisfaction with his or her past life, or despair and disgust over past failures. More recent workers have proposed an anti-stage theory of ageing, where personality, development, and adjustment are affected by historical events throughout life.

Most studies have reported relative stability of personality traits from adulthood into late life. When personality changes occur, they appear to be related to losses, particularly those involving health and social support systems. Some studies have reported sex differences in personality in older age, men tending to become more affiliative and nurturing and women tending to become more individualistic and more aggressive as they become older.

Further reading

Busse EW (2002). General theories of aging. In: *Principles and practice of geriatric psychiatry*, 2nd edn (ed. JRM Copeland, MT Abou-Saleh, and DG Blazer), pp. 19–22. Chichester, John Wiley.

Blanchflower DG. Unhappiness and age. J Econ Behav Organ. 2020;176:461–488.

Chaib S, Tchkonia T, Kirkland JL. Cellular senescence and senolytics: the path to the clinic. Nature Medicine. 2022 2022/08/01;28(8):1556–1568.

da Costa JP, Vitorino R, Silva GM, et al. A synopsis on aging—Theories, mechanisms and future prospects. Ageing Res Rev. 2016 Aug;29:90–112.

Chapter 2

Dementia

Introduction

- Dementia describes a clinical syndrome which has three manifestations: cognitive, neuropsychiatric, and in activities of daily living (ADLs). A traditional definition of dementia is useful to bear in mind (e.g. an acquired global impairment of higher mental functions without impairment of consciousness). This distinguishes it from learning disability (i.e. it is acquired), emphasizes the global nature of the symptoms (as opposed to an isolated amnesia), and distinguishes it from delirium (which is characterized by clouding of consciousness).
- The expression of the syndrome of dementia, therefore, can be conveniently described in these three main areas, with an emphasis on one or more of the clinical features indicating the cause (e.g. slow onset of cognitive loss in AD compared with vascular dementia (VaD), florid psychiatric symptoms in DLB).
- As a syndrome, the term 'dementia' is similar to describing 'liver failure' or 'heart failure'. Recently, some commentators have suggested that we should return to the older concept of 'brain failure' rather than dementia as it more accurately defines the clinical syndrome, but the overwhelming negative connotations of 'brain failure' make this unlikely in practice.
- Like many syndromes, dementia can be driven by a wide variety of diseases, from the common (Alzheimer's disease, vascular dementia, dementia with Lewy bodies) to the rare (e.g. prion diseases).

The syndrome of dementia

Cognitive deficits
  - Amnesia, dysphasia, agnosia, apraxia
- Neuropsychiatric features
  - Behavioural and psychological symptoms of dementia (BPSD)
  - Psychiatric symptoms
  - Behavioural disturbances
- Activities of daily living
  - Instrumental
  - Basic

The manifestation of dementia

The manifestation of the clinical syndrome of dementia can be divided into three parts:

- First, cognitive deficits, consisting of: amnesia (loss of memory); dysphasia (either a receptive aphasia or expressive dysphasia, the latter being more apparent in conversation, and nominal dysphasia tested by direct questioning of naming of objects); apraxia (the inability to carry out tasks despite intact sensory and motor nervous systems, manifest in dementia most usually by an inability to dress, often shown by putting on a shirt or coat back to front, or the inability to use a knife and fork correctly); and agnosia (the inability to recognize things such as one's own mirror reflection or a family member—remember, this is different from forgetting someone's name).
- Second, a neuropsychiatric component with symptoms such as psychiatric disturbances and behavioural disorders (also known as behavioural and psychological symptoms of dementia, BPSD) which are present in a substantial proportion of patients. The commonest are (approximate frequencies in brackets): depression (up to 66% at some point during their dementia); paranoid ideation (30%); misidentifications (usually based on agnosia, 20%); hallucinations (most commonly auditory, suspect an intercurrent delirium or dementia with Lewy bodies if persistent visual hallucinations are present, 15%); aggression (20%); wandering (20%). An alternative way of describing these features appears in Fig. 2.1.
- Third, deficits in ADLs. Towards the later stages of dementia these are manifest by obvious problems in dressing, eating, and going to the toilet. In the early stages they may be manifest by a failure to wash or dress to a person's usual standard, or by difficulties in managing complex but everyday tasks like using television remote controls or household appliances. In people living alone, neglect of diet can lead to weight loss, and neglect of household tasks may lead to comments about cleanliness of the house.

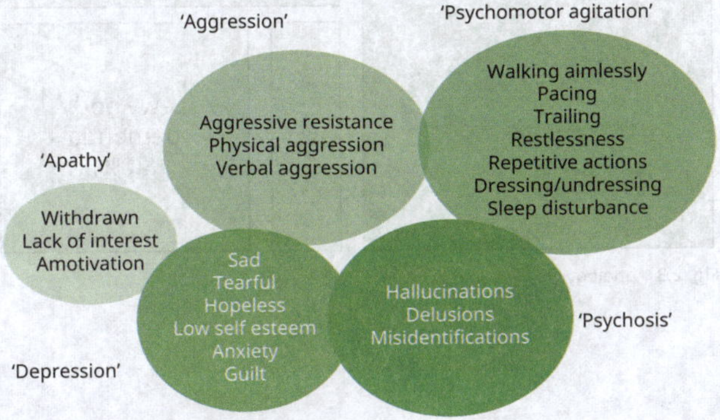

Fig. 2.1 Neuropsychiatric syndromes in dementia.
Source: Data from McShane R. What Are the Syndromes of Behavioral and Psychological Symptoms of Dementia? *Int Psychogeriatr 2000*; 12 (Supp1): 147–153.

Diagnosis and differential diagnosis

The diagnosis of dementia is a two-stage process. First, the diagnosis of dementia, as a clinical syndrome, and second, the elucidation of the aetiology of the dementia. The main differential diagnoses of dementia and its aetiology are summarized in Figs 2.2 and 2.3.

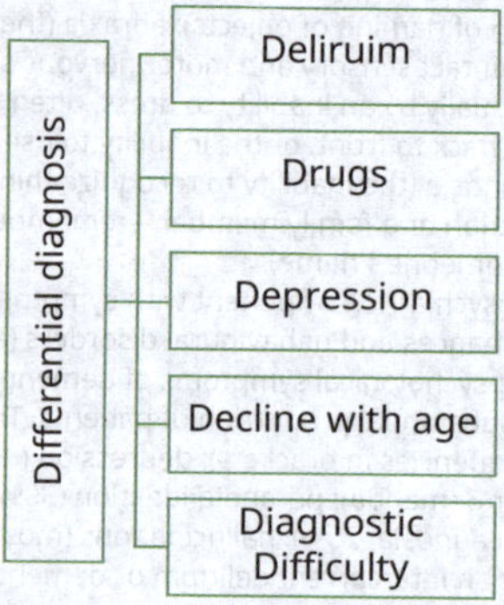

Fig. 2.2 Differential diagnosis.

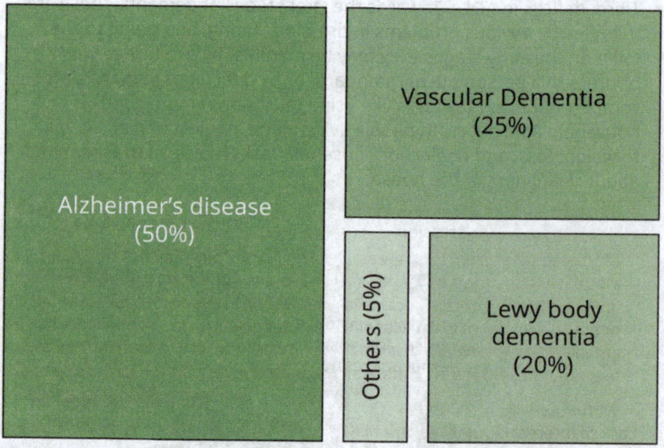

Fig. 2.3 Aetiology.

Differential diagnosis of dementia: depression

Depression

The symptoms of depression can be similar to those of dementia and the term 'pseudodementia' has been used to describe people in whom the presenting symptoms are highly suggestive of a dementia but whose primary diagnosis, after investigation and treatment, is depression (Table 2.1). Patients with depression and no evidence of dementia may also present with self-neglect and loss of interest and may perform poorly on tests of cognitive function, often giving depressive 'don't know' answers to questions rather than providing an incorrect answer. The diagnosis of depression can usually be reached if patients are questioned about their mood, and symptoms such as diurnal mood variation, poor appetite, early morning wakening, poor concentration, anergia, negative thoughts about the future and their own self-worth. Crying (or at least the feeling that a person wants to cry but is unable to do so) is a sensitive measure of depressed mood. Older people may not complain of low mood but will admit to experiencing a loss of pleasure (anhedonia) and to giving up their interests over and above what might be normally expected for an older person. Failure to enjoy the presence of loved ones such as grandchildren is a sensitive indicator of significant depression.

Table 2.1 Pseudodementia and dementia—characteristic features

	Pseudodementia	Dementia
Aetiology	Mood disorder, or other reversible psychiatric cause which includes mood symptoms.	Neurodegeneration.
Clinical features	Symptoms present and evolve more quickly than in dementia. Often a trigger event prior to symptoms.	Gradual progression of symptoms, often over years.
	Psychological, cognitive, and biological symptoms of depression. Any psychotic symptoms are mood congruent.	Behavioural and psychological symptoms of dementia (BPSD) may include delusions of theft or infidelity.
	Family history of mood disorder likely.	
Function	May have motivational impairment, but able to perform activities of daily living.	As dementia progresses, unable to perform activities of daily living even if motivated to do so.
Cognitive testing	Cognitive testing improves as mood symptoms resolve.	Consistent, progressive decline in scores.
	Patients find testing effortful and may lack motivation.	Cognitive impairment despite trying to complete tasks.
Neuroimaging	No disproportionate cerebral atrophy or other organic cause for memory symptoms.	Likely to show characteristic changes depending on subtype, e.g. hippocampal atrophy in Alzheimer's disease.
Prognosis	Symptom resolution, but recurrence possible.	Symptoms progress with time.
Management	Psychosocial support, talking therapy and antidepressant medication.	Consider care requirements, cholinesterase inhibitors, memantine.
	Next-line pharmacological options and ECT in cases of treatment resistance.	ECT inappropriate.

Differential diagnosis of dementia: mild cognitive impairment

Clinical features

In clinic, patients are often encountered who report memory or other cognitive problems, and show deficits on cognitive testing, but are not functionally impaired. There is a number of terms to describe this type of decline of memory and executive function and the implications this has for the individual. 'Mild cognitive impairment' (MCI) is the term which has stuck and is the most widely used. It describes the clinical situation where a person complains of memory problems which is corroborated by others, and where there is objective evidence of cognitive dysfunction, but not sufficient evidence to meet a diagnosis of a dementia syndrome. In particular, patients will not meet the functional impairment criteria required for a dementia diagnosis.

Diagnosis

The diagnostic criteria for MCI have been formalized by Petersen and colleagues[1] thus:

- Cognitive complaint, usually memory.
- Normal general cognitive function, i.e. cognitive screening test in normal range for age.
- 1.5 standard deviations below age-appropriate norms on memory tests or memory component of other cognitive tests (tests determined by clinician judgement).
- ADLs not significantly affected.
- Not meeting DSM dementia criteria, i.e. impairments not sufficient to impair professional and social activities.

Neuropsychological instruments can be used to screen for MCI; the MoCA, the test developed for the Consortium to Establish a Registry for Alzheimer's Disease (CERAD), Addenbrooke's Cognitive Examination – Revised (ACE-R), and the Quick Mild Cognitive Impairment (Qmci) screen have similar diagnostic accuracy, whereas the MMSE has the lowest sensitivity. The Memory Alteration Test has the highest sensitivity and equivalent specificity to the other tests.

The concept of MCI can be further subdivided into amnestic MCI (aMCI) and non-amnestic MCI (naMCI), referring to patients who complain about cognition, are not demented, but who show impairment on testing on a non-memory domain of cognition (see Fig. 2.4). The related term of 'mild behavioural impairment' (MBI) has also been used to describe early behavioural and neuropsychiatric symptoms suggestive of dementia which are often missed or overlooked. These can be captured using scales such as the Mild Behavioural Impairment Checklist (MBI-C), the Frontal Behavioural Inventory (FBI), or the Neuropsychiatric Inventory Questionnaire (NPI-Q). The concept of subjective cognitive decline (SCD) describes the situation of a patient presenting with subjectively impaired memory but normal neuropsychological testing and no impairment in their ADLs.

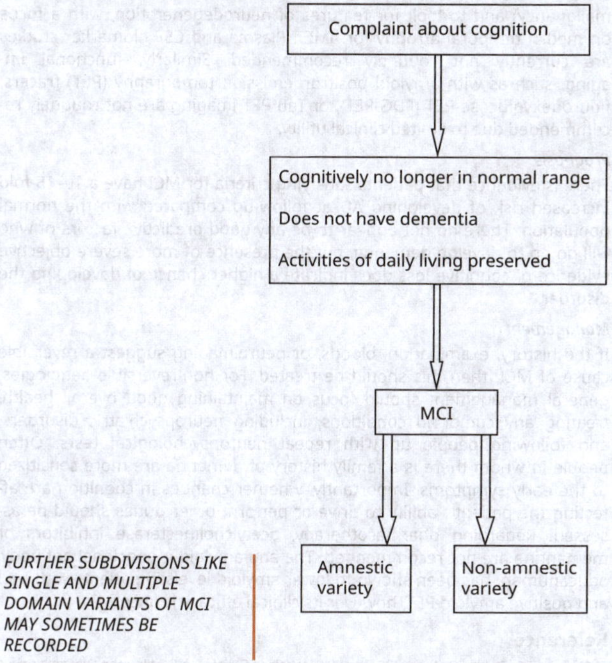

Fig. 2.4 Steps in arriving at a diagnosis of Mild Cognitive Impairment (MCI).

Neuropathology

MCI can be thought of as a precursor state to neurodegeneration, with neuropathological evidence in MCI samples suggesting that the underlying process is mainly Alzheimer's disease (AD) pathology affecting the medial temporal lobes. Additionally, vascular insults and other neurodegenerative processes may be responsible. Postmortem brain studies suggest that central cholinergic function is relatively preserved at earlier disease stages in AD.

Epidemiology

A recent systematic review suggests that MCI prevalence is 6.7% for ages 60–64, rising to 25.2% for ages 80–84. Other studies suggest an overall prevalence of 13–18 % for those over 50.

Investigations

Workup should be similar to dementia, to exclude reversible causes and identify a possible aetiology. This should include routine bloods (especially for B12 and thyroid function tests) and MRI to rule out structural causes (e.g. normal pressure hydrocephalus, subdural haematoma, neurological malignancy) and to look for features of neurodegeneration, with a focus on medial temporal atrophy for aMCI. Plasma and CSF biomarker studies are currently not routinely recommended. Similarly, functional imaging, such as with amyloid positron emission tomography (PET) tracers, flourodexyglucose-PET (FDG-PET), or Tau PET imaging are not routinely recommended due to limited clinical utility.

Prognosis

There is evidence that patients satisfying criteria for MCI have a 10–15-fold increased risk of developing AD at follow-up compared with the normal population. There do not appear to be any good predictive factors of who will go on to develop dementia, but the presence of more severe objective evidence of cognitive loss does indicate a higher chance of developing the disorder.

Management

If the history, examination, bloods, or neuroimaging suggest a reversible cause of MCI, then this should be treated. For non-reversible aetiologies, general management should focus on maintaining good overall health, treating any comorbid conditions, including neuropsychiatric disorders, and following people up with repeat neuropsychological tests. Often people in whom there is a family history of dementia are more sensitized to the early symptoms. Importantly, whether changes in cognition are affecting the patient's ability to drive or perform other duties should be assessed. Regarding pharmacotherapy, acetylcholinesterase inhibitors or memantine are not recommended. The anti-amyloid monoclonal antibody, aducanumab, has been shown to lower amyloid levels in patients with MCI and positive amyloid PET, however its clinical efficacy is uncertain.

Reference

1. Petersen RC, Smith GE, Waring SC, Ivnik RJ, Tangalos EG, Kokmen E. Mild cognitive impairment: Clinical characterization and outcome. Arch Neurol. 1999;56(3):303–308.

Differential diagnosis of dementia: other differentials

Delirium

One of the most important differential diagnoses of dementia is delirium (also called 'acute confusional state'). Delirium (see Chapter 3 for a detailed account) is recognised by the presence of marked fluctuations in the clinical picture of the patient: a change over a day may cause relatives and even staff to mistakenly [illegible] dementia [illegible] exercised by the patient [illegible] is characteristically associated with impaired concentration, poor attention, overarousal, changes in behaviour [illegible], and perceptual abnormalities such as visual hallucinations. Clouding of consciousness was previously the hallmark by which delirium was diagnosed but this is a difficult sign to detect and disturbance of attention and concentration [illegible] is used as a proxy measure. It can be difficult to differentiate between delirium and a dementia [illegible] fluctuating [illegible] DLB. A clear history of [illegible] onset [illegible] precipitating [illegible] will usually [illegible] the [illegible].

Drugs

A number of drugs can give rise to symptoms of dementia. A proper drug history can usually pick up drugs which have been prescribed and which can adversely affect cognitive function. Drugs with [illegible] anticholinergic side effects are particularly commonly given to older people and cause [illegible] cognitive impairment. Benzodiazepines may [illegible] older people and [illegible] cognitive [illegible] may produce cognitive impairment [illegible] In particular, new [illegible] and [illegible] agonists can precipitate [illegible] psychiatric changes.

Diagnostic difficulty

The cornerstone of an accurate diagnosis of dementia is a history from a reliable informant and [illegible] there is always doubt. People with severe sensory impairment (visual and/or hearing) [illegible] because of communication difficulties [illegible] individuals who have [illegible] which can be hard to characterise. [illegible] in the diagnosis of dementia in individuals with [illegible] particularly given the [illegible] life expectancy [illegible] with learning disability, especially Down syndrome [illegible] changes consistent with AD.

Differential diagnosis at diagnostic stage

The four primary dementia syndromes are AD, vascular cognitive impairment (VCI), Lewy body dementia (LBD), and frontotemporal dementia (FTD).

Other causes of dementia include Huntington's disease, normal pressure hydrocephalus, [illegible] vitamin B_{12} deficiency, [illegible] alcohol-related dementia, Creutzfeldt–Jakob disease, and progressive supranuclear palsy. [illegible] transient global amnesia (TGA).

Differential diagnosis of dementia: other differentials

Delirium

One of the most important differential diagnoses of dementia is delirium (also called colloquially a confusional state)[1]. Delirium (see Chapter 3 for a detailed account) can be recognized by the presence of marked fluctuations in the clinical picture of the patient (a change over a day may cause relatives and even staff to mistakenly suppose a degree of control is being exercised by the patient) and is characteristically associated with impaired concentration, poor attention, overarousal, changes in behaviour, fearful affect, and perceptual abnormalities such as visual hallucinations. Clouding of consciousness was previously the hallmark by which delirium was diagnosed but it is a difficult sign to detect and disorders of attention and concentration tend to be used as proxy measures. It can be difficult to differentiate between delirium and a dementia characterized by fluctuating cognitive performance such as VaD or DLB. A clear history of abrupt onset, drug or illness precipitants, and quick improvement in the syndrome will usually decide the matter.

Drugs

A number of drugs can give rise to symptoms of dementia. A proper drug history can usually pick up drugs which have been prescribed and which can adversely affect cognitive function. Drugs which cause anticholinergic side effects are particularly commonly given to older people and can exacerbate cognitive impairment. Benzodiazepines may oversedate older people and diminish cognitive performance. Antiparkinsonian treatments may cause profound cognitive impairment and features of delirium and/or psychosis. In particular, new initiations of dopamine agonists can precipitate dramatic psychiatric changes.

Diagnostic difficulty

The cornerstone of an accurate diagnosis of dementia is a history from a reliable informant and if there is none available there is always doubt. People with severe sensory impairment (visual and/or hearing) can provide a challenge because of communication difficulties and (although seen much less often now) individuals who have been institutionalized for many years can have behaviours which can be hard to characterize. Specialist expertise in the diagnosis of dementia in individuals with learning disability is often needed; particularly given the greater life expectancy among people with learning disability, especially Down's syndrome (most older Down's syndrome patients manifest changes consistent with AD).

Differential diagnosis: diagnostic sieve

The four primary dementia syndromes are AD, vascular cognitive impairment (VCI), Lewy body dementia (LBD) and frontotemporal dementia (FTD).

Other causes of dementia include Huntington's disease, neurosyphilis, normal pressure hydrocephalus, hypothyroidism, vitamin B_{12} deficiency, head trauma, alcohol-related dementias, Creutzfeldt–Jakob disease and progressive supranuclear palsy. Acute transient amnesia can sometimes be secondary to transient global amnesia (TGA).

Cortical dementias

- Alzheimer's disease (AD).
- Frontal lobe degeneration (FTD, Pick's disease).

Subcortical dementias

- Extrapyramidal syndrome:
  - Parkinson's disease
  - Huntington's disease
  - Progressive supranuclear palsy
  - Wilson's disease
  - Spinocerebellar degenerations
  - Idiopathic and basal ganglia calcification.
- Hydrocephalus.
- Dementia syndrome in depression.
- White matter diseases:
  - Multiple sclerosis.
  - HIV encephalopathy.

Vascular

- Lacunar state.
- Binswanger's disease.
- Reversible posterior leukoencephalopathy syndrome (RPLS).
- Cerebral venous sinus thrombosis.
- Cerebral amyloid angiopathy (CAA), amyloid beta-related angiitis (ABRA).

Dementias with combined cortical and subcortical dysfunction

- Multi-infarct dementias.

Infectious diseases

- Slow virus dementias and general paralysis.
- Whipple's disease.

Toxic and metabolic encephalopathies

- Systemic illnesses.
- Endocrinopathies.
- Deficiency states.
- Drug intoxications.
- Heavy metal exposure.
- Industrial dementias.

Miscellaneous dementia syndromes

- Autoimmune encephalitis.
- Post-traumatic.
- Post-anoxic.
- Neoplastic.

Reference

1. From Cummings JL and Benson DF (1992). Dementia: A clinical approach, 2nd edn. London, Butterworth Heinemann.

Signs and symptoms of dementia

People with the symptoms of dementia may present to specialist services for help at various stages of their illness—in the past, this was usually when the symptoms were of moderate severity and had started to impair day-to-day activities. The advent of memory clinics and the overall increase in the publicity surrounding dementia and AD has undoubtedly prompted people to come forward earlier for investigation and treatment, and early diagnosis and access to treatment is now an identified priority. By the moderate and severe stages the patient will be usually unable to give an accurate history, and indeed may deny any difficulties. A collateral history should be obtained from anyone available, preferably a family member. Although the symptoms may appear to have had a sudden onset, perhaps coinciding with the death of a spouse or a move from a familiar neighbourhood, such an impression may have merely brought the condition to the notice of others. Support of the patient by a spouse or other caregiver can minimize problems that become evident to others only after a bereavement. A good history from a close relative usually describes the true sequence of events. Failing cognitive function can be minimized by adherence to rigid routines that are disrupted when the patient moves away from familiar surroundings, so a strong clue is family reporting the patient suddenly struggling on a holiday or visit to relatives.

The overall course of AD is usually steadily and smoothly progressive with death following usually within 5–7 years when the onset is in later life. Figure 2.5 shows the changes that occur during the course of dementia. Theoretically, there may be an initiating factor, such as a genetic predisposition to the illness, followed by a promoting event such as a head injury at some point before the onset of the first symptoms. Often, in retrospect, emotional changes can be one of the first noticeable alterations. Problems with cognitive function supervene shortly after with deterioration following an S-shaped decline (relatively fast deterioration in the middle stages), with problems in ADLs and then deterioration in behaviour (this is obviously an oversimplification of a more complex process).

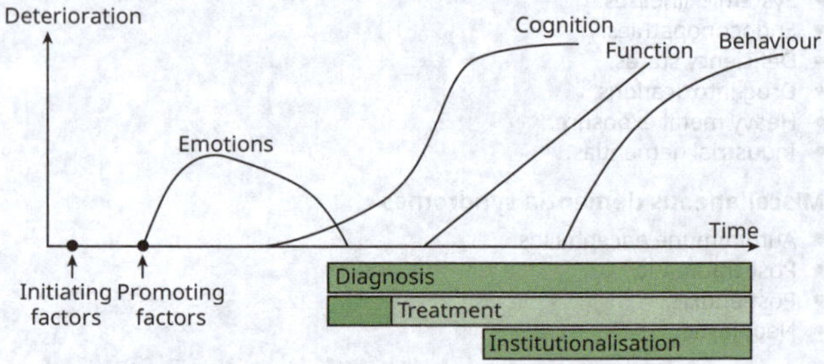

Fig. 2.5 The natural history of dementia.

History

- Begin by noting the patient's age, handedness, occupation, and key medical background, together with the presenting complaint (PC) including time course and progression. For example, 'a 75-year-old, right-handed ex-builder with a background of hypertension presents with difficulties with word finding which came on after a stroke and persisted ever since'.
- The single most helpful investigation is obtaining a history from the patient together with information from informants, from whom it is particularly important to obtain a history of the temporal sequence of events since the onset of the problems. These will include members of the patient's family and close friends and other professionals involved with the patient. The patient's general practitioner (GP) or primary care physician is obviously a valuable source of information about the patient's family history, past medical and personal history, pre-morbid personality, social circumstances, and dynamics of family relationships.
- Discussion with an informant will usually establish the onset and duration of the presenting problem. Difficulties with memory and changes in personality are usual. Problems encountered with hobbies such as following a complicated knitting pattern or playing bridge may be the first change noted. Difficulties may have become apparent after a sudden alteration in circumstances such as the death of a spouse. The course of the illness is also of importance in distinguishing between VaD and AD. A detailed account of the difficulties that patients experience in their ADLs is important with due deference paid to preserved abilities.
- Evidence of memory impairment can be obtained from the patient telling the same story or asking the same questions during the interview as well as from specific questions about whether the patient forgets, unless reminded, family anniversaries or important appointments. Reports of episodes where patients become lost are also important. Language difficulties may be apparent during the interview but are often elicited only on direct questioning. Evidence of dyspraxia can be obtained by judging the patient's ability to use a knife and fork and to dress. Changes in personal habits or interactions with family or friends may indicate a change in personality. Evidence of hallucinations or delusions can also be obtained from family members who may describe the situation when the patient appears to talk to someone when there is no-one there, to see things when no-one else can, or to have odd ideas, e.g. accusing others of stealing from him or her or of not being who they claim.
- Medical history may be of aetiological importance, such as a family history of dementia or vascular risk factors such as hypertension, diabetes, ischaemic heart disease, or stroke/transient ischaemic attack (TIA).

Mental state examination in dementia

The discipline of adhering to the traditional headings in the mental state examination is important in a logical assessment. Bear in mind that it can be as important how a person says something as exactly what they say. This can often be apparent when a relative interrupts to correct what is in reality a minor point of fact.

Appearance and behaviour

- Disinhibited or inappropriate behaviour is often apparent and worthy of note, and guarded or irritable behaviour may indicate paranoid ideas or personality change. Clouding of consciousness is an important clinical sign in differentiating between a delirium and a dementia but very difficult to detect unless a person obviously has wandering attention and even drowsiness. Never forget to make a visual physical assessment, and the easy recognition of pallor, jaundice, or even finger clubbing is invariably helpful as well as reinforcing the medical training of the assessor. Overt signs of depression, such as agitation or psychomotor retardation, may be apparent at interview. MBI can precede neurodegeneration.

Speech

- Evidence of dysphasia or dysarthria can be obvious. Other abnormalities include perseveration (when the patient continues to give the answer to the previous question in response to new questions), pallilalia (when the last word of an answer is repeated with increasing frequency), logoclonia (when the last syllable is repeated), and logorrhoea (a meaningless outpouring of words). The patient may echo the examiner's speech (echolalia) or actions (echopraxia). These signs are rarely seen but never forgotten. In dementia, speech may more often be fluent but somewhat banal, indicating paucity of content. Social skills may be superficially preserved but varying questions will reveal limited and repetitive responses.

Mood

- Mood disturbances are often found in association with dementia and can be the presenting feature. Objective evidence of agitation, anxiety, irritability, or low mood should be noted. Subjective symptoms of depression are less likely to be forthcoming but should be sought. Comment on mood constancy and congruency.

Thought content

- The content of thought is often impoverished in dementia but careful questioning may reveal the presence of delusions or depressive ideas and the patient may elaborate on psychotic experiences. Delusional misidentifications are particularly striking where a person reports having two of something, such as a spouse or home. Note whether there is formal thought disorder, paranoid, morbid, obsessive, or anxious thoughts. In dementia, mundane delusions, for example that someone has stolen their glasses or money, are common.

Perceptions

- Some patients may be hallucinating at interview but as psychotic symptoms are common in dementia they should be inquired about in all patients by a non-directive question such as 'Does your imagination play tricks on you?'

Cognition

- Traditionally, this was assessed using a number of unstructured questions covering the main domains of orientation to time and place (and often person, indicating the recognition of other people), attention (counting back from 20 to 1, or months of the year backwards), short- and long-term memory (immediate recall of a name and address, e.g. John Brown, 42 Church Street, Bedford; and autobiographical details such as the name of the person's first school), language (naming objects), and praxis (drawing a three-dimensional cube).
- Standardized tests such as the MoCA are helpful in establishing whether a cognitive deficit exists. Their advantages are that they can be repeated to show change over time and give a quantified and recognized measure of cognitive function. The disadvantage is that they have encouraged a formulaic approach to the assessment of cognition. A MoCA of 26 and above is considered normal, and age-adjusted cutoffs are available. However, some patients have extensive educational backgrounds, or will report that the usual, brief instruments used in clinic have not captured the change in cognition which they are experiencing. In these instances, careful exploration of the phenomenology of the patient's symptoms combined with the use of a more detailed neuropsychological test, such as the ACE-R-III, can help to pinpoint subtle problems. The Frontal Assessment Battery (FAB) is an example of an easily administered bedside test for frontal functions. Further details of assessment instruments are provided later.

Physical examination and investigation

Physical examination includes a search for the signs of conditions known to cause dementia. Blood pressure should be measured. Assessment of vision and hearing is important, as exacerbating factors. A neurological examination will detect focal neurological signs that are more commonly found in VaDs, the presence of primitive reflexes that are found in advanced dementia and may reveal parkinsonian signs in DLB.

Further investigations should be carried out for everyone in whom a dementia is suspected. In the past, tests were directed towards what were considered 'reversible' or 'potentially reversible' dementias, and it was standard teaching to test for vitamin B_{12} and folate and thyroid dysfunction in case one missed a treatable, i.e. reversible, dementia. Now, these investigations should be directed as much to identifying comorbid conditions which need and merit treatment in their own right, i.e. a person with VaD who has a lowish vitamin B_{12} level should have that treated not so much in the expectation that the dementia will be reversed but that a comorbidity will be treated in the same way that it would be if found in a person free from dementia.

Debate inevitably surrounds which screening tests are necessary, the argument being that the low yield makes them superfluous. A standard screen will usually include a full blood count, (alcohol-related dementia), erythrocyte sedimentation rate (ESR) (or C-reactive protein (CRP), inflammatory disease), vitamin B_{12} and folate (vitamin B_{12} and folate deficiency), urea and electrolytes (U&E) (metabolic disorders), calcium and phosphates (parathyroid disorder), syphilis serology (general paresis of the insane), HIV testing where appropriate (acquired immune deficiency syndrome dementia), chest X-ray, and ECG as indicated by abnormalities on clinical examination. Lumbar puncture is indicated if there is any evidence of encephalitis.

Potentially reversible causes of dementia are found in around 10% of people investigated, but only a fraction of these completely reverse with treatment of a comorbid condition although more will partially respond to treatment. The commonest causes are: drugs, depression, metabolic causes, thyroid disease, vitamin B_{12} deficiency, calcium disturbance, liver disease, normal pressure hydrocephalus, subdural haematoma, and neoplasm.

Dementia screen

- Always:
  - Full blood count
  - U&E
  - Thyroid function tests
  - Liver function tests
  - Vitamin B_{12}
  - Folate
  - ESR or CRP
  - Blood glucose
- Sometimes (when clinically indicated):
  - Syphilis serology
  - HIV testing
  - Calcium screen
  - Chest X-ray
  - ECG
  - Autoimmune encephalitis screen (e.g. Anti-NMDA, VGKC, LGI1, CASPR2, Glycine-R, GABA-B, AMPA-R, anti-neuronal, anti-nuclear)

Imaging in dementia

Neuroimaging is a routine part of diagnosis for neurocognitive disorders and often helpful in the differential of psychiatric symptoms in old age psychiatry. This differential includes structural brain lesions such as tumours (primary or secondary), cerebral infarctions, subdural or extradural haematomas, cerebral abscess, and normal pressure hydrocephalus. Whilst reporting on these scans is the province of the radiologist, some background understanding helps with deciding when requesting imaging is appropriate, what to ask for, how to understand the basics of the neuroradiologist's report, and with explaining the diagnosis to patients and relatives.

MRI is often used for patients presenting with cognitive or neuropsychiatric symptoms. As a reminder, MRI can be T1 weighted ('anatomical') versus T2 (CSF bright). The two most widely used scoring systems in dementia which may be encountered on radiology reports are the medial temporal lobe atrophy (MTA) score for AD, and the Fazekas score for white matter hyperintensities (WMHs), for VaD.

Medial Temporal lobe Atrophy (MTA) score

The MTA score indicates the severity of volume loss in the hippocampus from a score of 0 (no atrophy) to 4 (severe atrophy) (see Fig. 2.6). If under age 75, a score of 2 or more is abnormal, if over 75, 3 or more is considered abnormal. The T1 weighted images below demonstrate this for each score, which is based on the choroid fissure, temporal horn, and the height of the hippocampal formation

- MTA score 0: no atrophy
- MTA score 1: only widening of choroid fissure
- MTA score 2: also widening of temporal horn of lateral ventricle

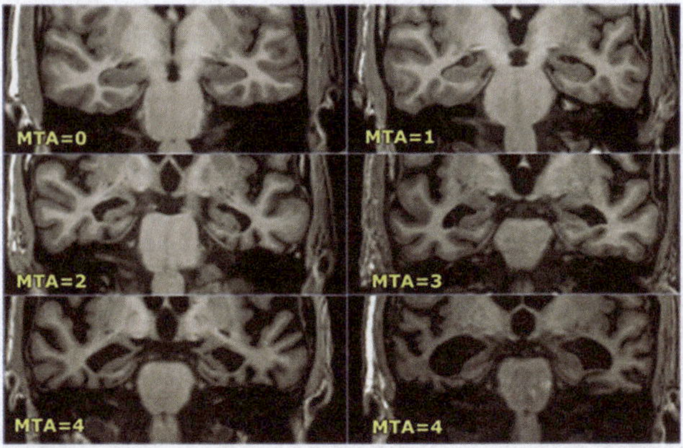

Fig. 2.6 Medial temporal atrophy score from 0 to 4.

Reproduced with kind permission of Prof. Frederik Barkhof, Professor of Neuroradiology, University College London (UCL). Available at https://radiologyassistant.nl/neuroradiology/dementia/role-of-mri

- MTA score 3: moderate loss of hippocampal volume (decrease in height)
- MTA score 4: severe volume loss of hippocampus

< 75 years: score 2 or more is abnormal, > 75 years: score 3 or more is abnormal.

Fazekas score

The Fazekas score for WMHs is useful with regards to VaD (see Fig. 2.7). The score runs from 0, no or a single punctate WMH lesion; to 1, indicating multiple punctate lesions; to 2, bridging of lesions; to 3, large, confluent WMH lesions.

- Fazekas 0: None or a single punctate WMH lesion
- Fazekas 1: Multiple punctate lesions
- Fazekas 2: Beginning confluency of lesions (bridging)
- Fazekas 3: Large confluent lesions

An approach to understanding MRI images in cognitive impairment

The following elements comprise a way of understanding an MRI image and its report (see Table 2.2). The radiologist will usually have reported on all

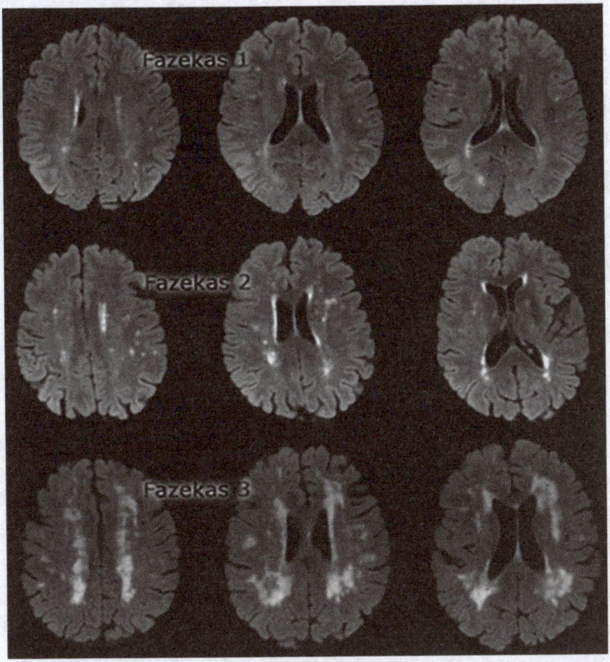

Fig. 2.7 Fazekas score from 1 to 3.
Reproduced with kind permission of Prof. Frederik Barkhof, Professor of Neuroradiology, UCL Available at https://radiologyassistant.nl/neuroradiology/dementia/role-of-mri

Table 2.2 MR atrophic findings for different dementia subtypes (AD, VaD, FTD)

	AD	VaD	FTD
Hippocampus	Severe	Mild to moderate	Moderate
Temporal lobe	Moderate to severe	Mild	Moderate to severe
Frontal lobe	-	Mild	Severe
Parietal lobe	Moderate to severe	Mild	-
Infarctions and WMHs	-	Moderate to severe	-

Source: data from Barkhof F. DementiaRole of MRI 2022. Available at https://radiologyassistant.nl/neuroradiology/dementia/role-of-mri

these elements, if relevant. Note: Lewy body dementia is not associated with specific lobar atrophic or WMH findings.

1. GCA (Pasquier)—scale for global cortical atrophy, which runs from 0 (none) to 3 (knife blade atrophy)
2. Temporal lobe: MTA-scale for medial temporal lobe atrophy
3. Parietal lobe: Koedam score for parietal atrophy (0 indicating none, 3 indicating severe parietal atrophy), which may be present in AD
4. Infarcts: Fazekas scale for white matter lesions and any comments on infarctions in key areas for cognition

Further reading

Barkhof F. Dementia—Role of MRI 2022. Available from https://radiologyassistant.nl/neuroradiology/dementia/role-of-mri[1]

Barkhof FF, Bastos-Leite A, Scheltens, P (2011). *Neuroimaging in dementia*. Heidelberg: Springer.

Functional imaging in dementia

[illegible]

Functional imaging in dementia

Advanced imaging and nuclear medicine techniques are useful when the diagnosis is unclear or to confirm a specific suspected diagnosis, e.g. Lewy body dementia. These imaging modalities allow us to assess different aspects of brain function rather than a simple assessment of structure (i.e. with structural MRI). Whilst not a nuclear medicine technique, an electroencephalogram (EEG) can also provide functional information about the brain.

Single-photon emission computed tomography (SPECT) and PET are both nuclear medicine techniques. SPECT has been used to assess brain perfusion, and PET to assess metabolic processes in the brain.

Radioisotopes are unstable forms of chemical elements which emit radiation to become more stable. This radiation can be detected by specialized cameras. Radiopharmaceuticals combine these radioisotopes with biologically active substances to probe physiological processes.

Single-photon emission computed tomography (SPECT)

- SPECT uses gamma ray-emitting radioisotopes. SPECT involves the administration of compounds that are distributed in the brain according to cerebral blood flow; in this way, a relative measure of cerebral activity can be assessed in different brain regions. Most commonly, SPECT investigations measure blood flow, e.g. perfusion hexamethylpropyleneamine oxime (HMPAO) SPECT. SPECT imaging can be useful as an adjunct to the diagnosis of dementia. Characteristic temporo-parietal hypoperfusion is seen in AD, frontal hypoperfusion is a hallmark finding in dementia of the frontal lobe type, and patchy deficits may indicate vascular cognitive impairment.
- Ligands for dopamine transporters have been developed which when used in SPECT imaging (DaTscans) are certainly helpful in distinguishing parkinsonian syndromes (including DLB and Parkinson's disease) from other syndromes which can cause tremor (benign essential tremor and AD).
- SPECT is more widely available and cheaper than PET, and has been used for longer

Positron emission tomography (PET)

- PET uses positron-emitting radioisotopes (see Figs 2.8–2.10). This provides a direct measure of cerebral metabolic activity and can be used to assess cerebral metabolism and cerebral receptors. Amyloid PET enables assessment of Aβ plaques *in vivo*.

Here is a suggested approach to thinking about using functional imaging, the exact sequence will depend on local expertise and availability of imaging modalities (Chételat et al. 2020):

- Start with a thorough clinical assessment. Consider structural MRI in the first instance if imaging is necessary. If AD pathology is suspected, and the clinical picture is clear, then no need for further imaging
- If AD pathology is suspected, but the case is atypical or the aetiology is complex, consider amyloid PET or FDG-PET
- If Lewy body dementia is suspected, consider a DaTscan or meta-iodobenzylguanidine (MIBG) cardiac scintigraphy.
- If a rarer dementia is suspected, consider an FDG-PET scan

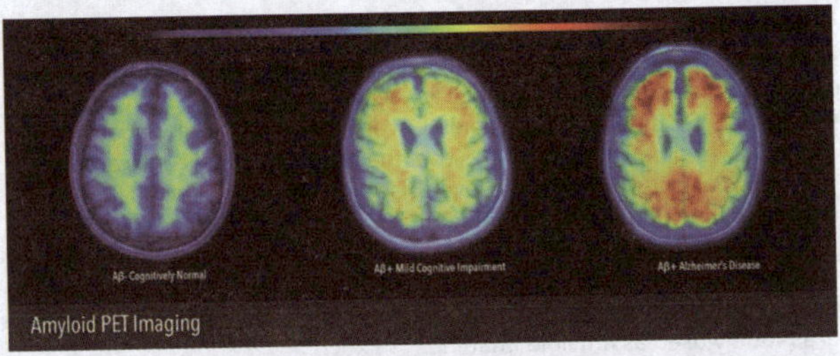

Fig. 2.8 Amyloid PET imaging in normal cognition, mild cognitive impairment patient and in Alzheimer's disease. Note the amount of amyloid in the brain does not necessarily correlate with symptoms.
Reproduced courtesy of William Jagust, Professor of Neuroscience, University of California, Berkeley

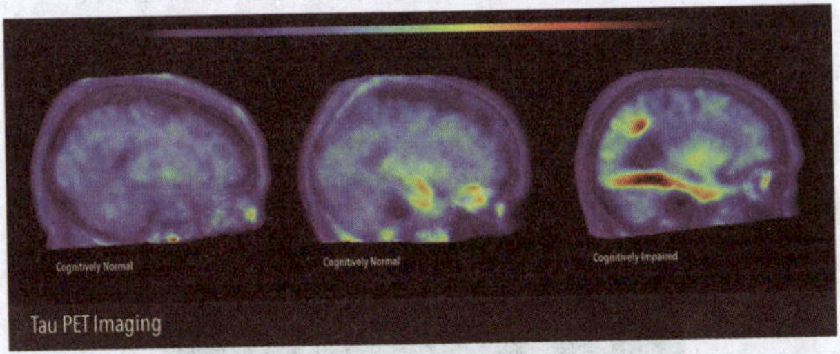

Fig. 2.9 Tau PET imaging example in normal cognition versus impairment.
Reproduced courtesy of William Jagust, Professor of Neuroscience, University of California, Berkeley

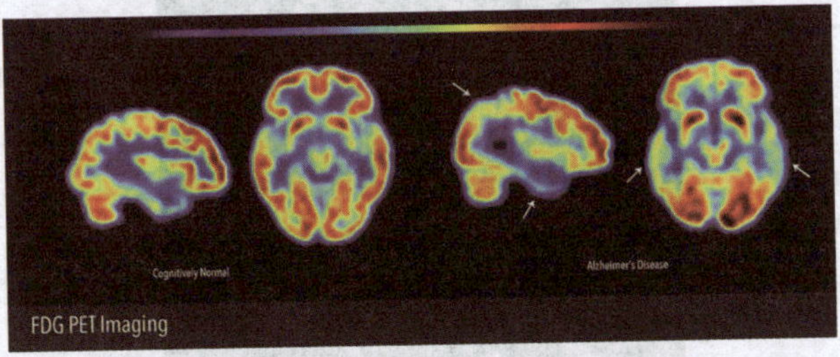

Fig. 2.10 FDG PET imaging in normal cognition and Alzheimer's disease. Arrows show areas of hypometabolism.
Reproduced courtesy of William Jagust, Professor of Neuroscience, University of California, Berkeley

Alzheimer's disease

- Flurodeoxyglucose-positron emission tomography (FDG-PET)
- Single photon emission CT (SPECT) (technetium-99)
- Amyloid PET: if negative, amyloid PET can rule out AD (high negative predictive value), however if positive, the results must take into account the clinical picture as amyloid levels rise with age in unaffected individuals. The most helpful use of amyloid PET is for clarifying the diagnosis in aetiologically mixed cases and for progressive MCI[2]. Amyloid PET has been used extensively in clinical trials of anti-amyloid agents.
- Tau PET imaging tracers allow for assessment of tauopathy, currently not as widely used as amyloid imaging.

Lewy body dementia (LBD)

- [^{123}I]FP-CIT (DaTscan) SPECT uses a radiotracer to bind to the dopamine transporter (see Figs 2.11–2.14). In LBD, there is a reduced striatal dopaminergic signal. Of note, several medications can interfere with radiotracer uptake which causes a false positive, and these should be stopped at least 5 half lives before the scan. Medications to be aware of are antidepressants (e.g. venlafaxine), amphetamines (e.g. methylphenidate), anti-anticholinergics, and anaesthetic drugs[3].
- [^{123}I]-MIBG cardiac scintigraphy. In LBD, degeneration occurs in postganglionic sympathetic nerves in the heart and patients show reduced uptake of the noradrenaline analogue metaiodobenzylguanidine (MIBG).

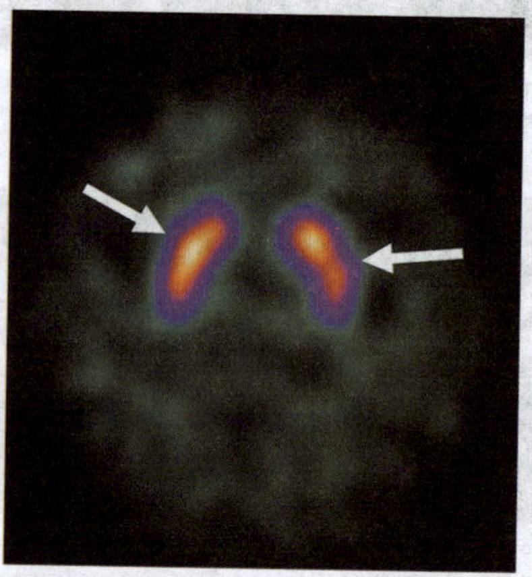

Fig. 2.11 Normal DaT scan. There is normal tracer uptake by both striata which demonstrate a comma shaped appearance (comma sign). There is no increased background cerebral uptake.

Reproduced courtesy of Dr Stefan Lazic, Consultant Radiologist, King's College Hospital NHS Foundation Trust

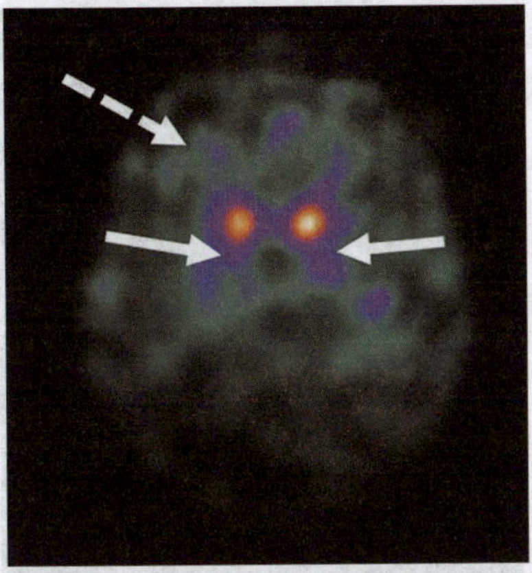

Fig. 2.12 Abnormal DaT scan suggesting Parkinsonian syndrome or idiopathic Parkinson's disease. There is severely reduced putaminal uptake bilaterally (solid arrows) with only some tracer uptake seen by the caudate heads ('dot' sign). There is increased background cerebral uptake (dashed arrow).

Reproduced courtesy of Dr Stefan Lazic, Consultant Radiologist, King's College Hospital NHS Foundation Trust

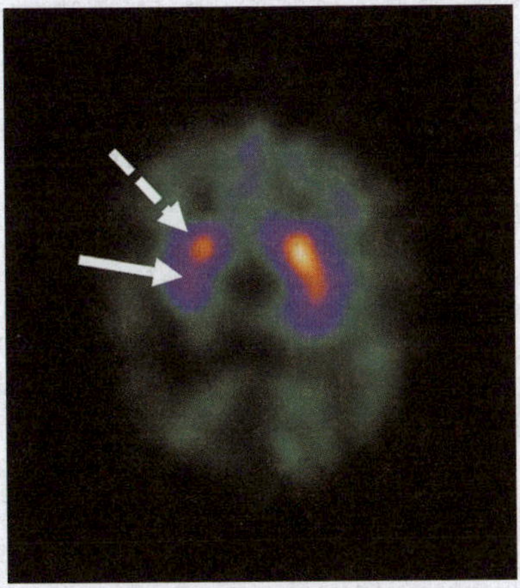

Fig. 2.13 Abnormal DaT scan suggesting vascular Parkinsonism. The left striatum shows normal tracer uptake, however the contralateral side is abnormal as evidenced by severely reduced uptake by the right putamen (solid arrow) and also reduced uptake by the right caudate head (dashed arrow).

Reproduced courtesy of Dr Stefan Lazic, Consultant Radiologist, King's College Hospital NHS Foundation Trust

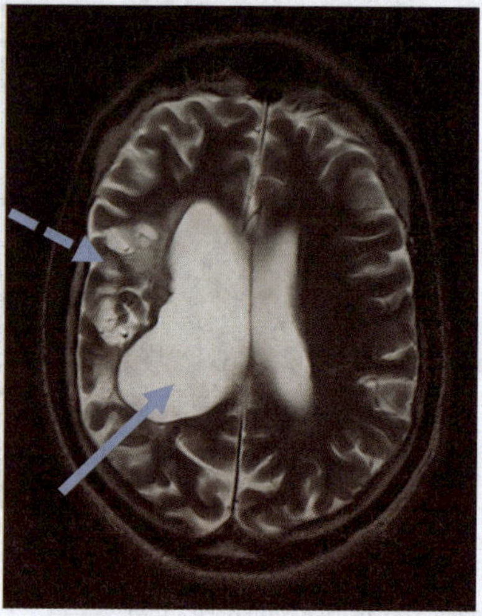

Fig. 2.14 MRI of the above patient (axial T2 slice) confirms a mature right middle cerebral artery territory infarct (which has involved the basal ganglia) as evidenced by enchaphalomalacia involving the right cerebral hemisphere (dashed arrow) with resultant ex-vacuo dilatation of the right lateral ventricle (solid arrow).

Reproduced courtesy of Dr Stefan Lazic, Consultant Radiologist, King's College Hospital NHS Foundation Trust

Frontotemporal dementia (FTD)

- Flurodeoxyglucose-positron emission tomography (FDG-PET)
- Single photon emission CT (SPECT) (technetium-99)

Electroencephalography (EEG)

- EEG can be useful in differentiating dementia from delirium. In normal ageing, the EEG has four predominant wave forms—delta (less than 4 Hz,) theta (4–7 Hz), alpha (8–13 Hz), and beta (14–30 Hz). In patients with severe dementia, EEG generally reveals significant abnormalities in terms of regular slow-wave activity. Generally, a relatively normal EEG in the presence of severe dementia is indicative of AD, whereas a very abnormal tracing with minimal clinical changes is associated with delirium. As the dementia progresses in AD there is slowing of the EEG tracing with decreased alpha and beta activity and increased, somewhat symmetrical, delta and theta waves.

Figures 2.15–2.19 depict the use of PET in distinguishing AD, frontotemporal dementia, and corticobasal degeneration.

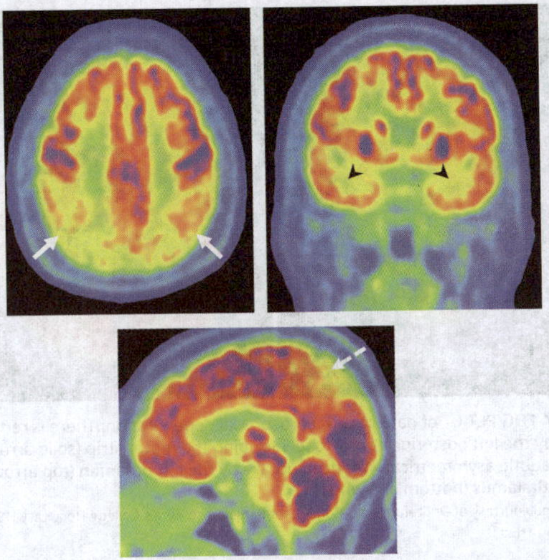

Fig. 2.15 FDG PET CT of a patient with Alzheimer's dementia. There is reduced tracer uptake by both parietal lobes (solid arrows) and both temporal lobes (arrowheads). There is also reduced tracer uptake by the cingulate gyrus (dashed arrow).
Reproduced courtesy of Dr Stefan Lazic, Consultant Radiologist, King's College Hospital NHS Foundation Trust

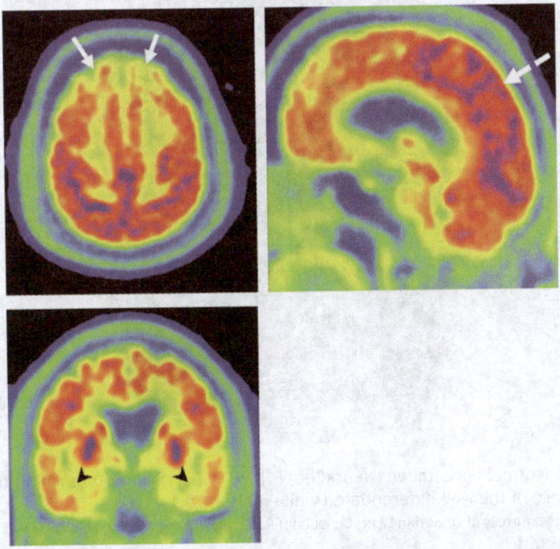

Fig. 2.16 FDG PET CT of a patient with frontotemporal dementia. There is reduced tracer uptake by both frontal lobes (solid arrows) and both temporal lobes (arrowheads). There is preserved uptake by the precuneus (dashed arrow).
Reproduced courtesy of Dr Stefan Lazic, Consultant Radiologist, King's College Hospital NHS Foundation Trust

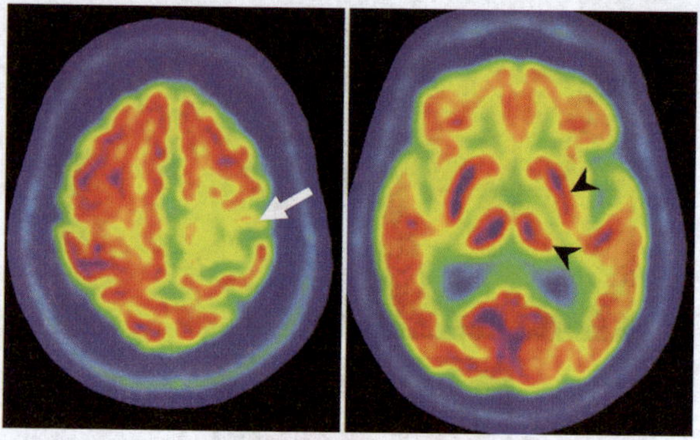

Fig. 2.17 FDG PET CT of patient with corticobasal degeneration. There is reduced uptake by the left posterior frontal lobe, including the motor strip (solid arrow) and there is subtle asymmetrically reduced uptake by the left putamen (top arrowhead) and left thalamus (bottom arrowhead).
Reproduced courtesy of Dr Stefan Lazic, Consultant Radiologist, King's College Hospital NHS Foundation Trust

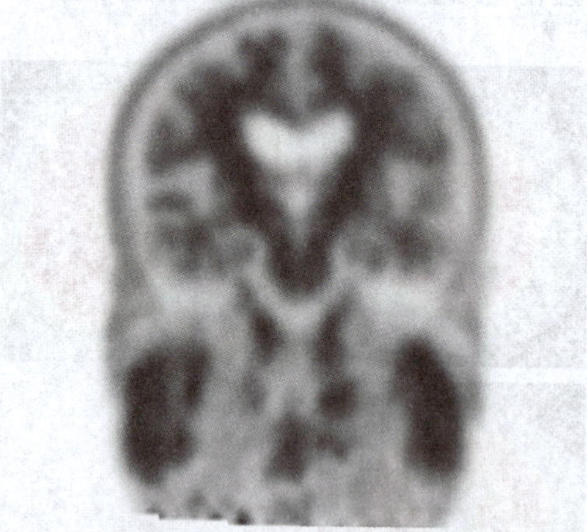

Fig. 2.18 Normal florbetaben (NeuraCeq) F18 PET CT showing a 'branching-tree' appearance of the well-differentiated white matter tracts.
Reproduced courtesy of Dr Stefan Lazic, Consultant Radiologist, King's College Hospital NHS Foundation Trust

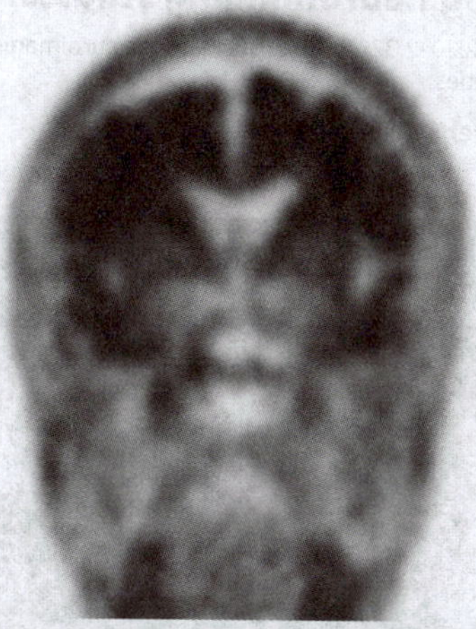

Fig. 2.19 Abnormal florbetaben (NeuraCeq) F18 PET CT showing a 'tree-in-bloom' appearance due to tracer uptake in the cerebral grey matter resulting in loss of grey-white matter differentiation. This indicates high levels of amyloid plaque deposition.

Reproduced courtesy of Dr Stefan Lazic, Consultant Radiologist, King's College Hospital NHS Foundation Trust

Further reading

Chételat G, Arbizu J, Barthel H, et al. Amyloid-PET and (18)F-FDG-PET in the diagnostic investigation of Alzheimer's disease and other dementias. Lancet Neurol. 2020 Nov;19(11):951–962.

Kolanko MA, Win Z, Loreto F, et al. Amyloid PET imaging in clinical practice. Pract Neurol. 2020 Dec;20(6):451–462.[2]

Kanani M-K, Gurunathan N. Misdiagnosis of dementia with Lewy bodies due to venlafaxine. Prog Neurol Psychiatry 2022;26(2):8–10.

Interpreting neuroimaging studies: cases

This section (Figs 2.20–2.32) consists of example neuroimaging studies using a range of modalities.

Case 1: Alzheimer's disease

See Figure 2.20

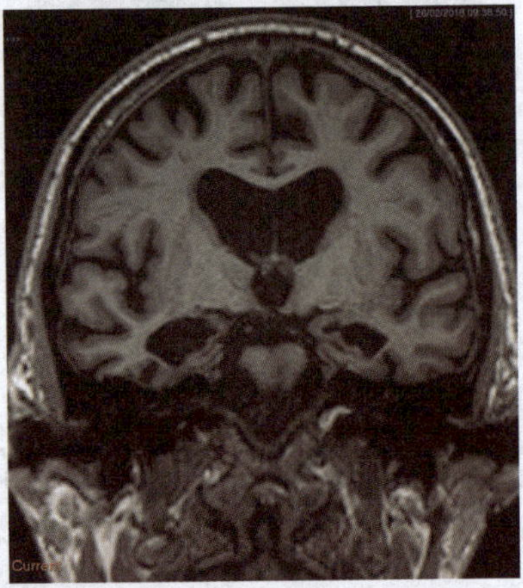

Fig. 2.20 Alzheimer's disease. T1-weighted coronal image of a patient with Alzheimer's dementia at the level of the hippocampal heads. There is marked bilateral mesial temporal volume loss, with severe hippocampal atrophy and expansion of the temporal horns of the lateral ventricles.

Reproduced courtesy of Dr Jack Garnham, Consultant Neuroradiologist, Imperial College Healthcare NHS Trust, and Dr Gemma Dawe, Consultant Neuroradiologist, Imperial College Healthcare NHS Trust

Case 2: Negative PET study, low cortical amyloid burden

See Figure 2.21

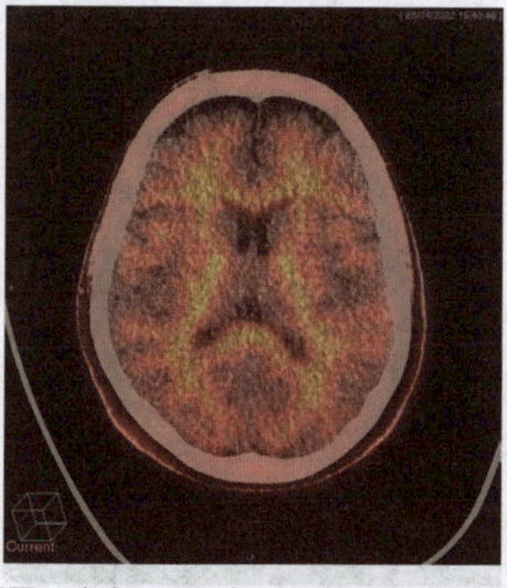

Fig. 2.21 Negative PET study, low cortical amyloid burden. Axial fused image from a florbetaben PET CT at the level of the lateral ventricles. There is normal tracer uptake in the white matter but no cortical tracer uptake, indicative of a low cortical amyloid burden. This is a negative study. Note the normal grey-white matter differentiation.
Reproduced courtesy of Dr Jack Garnham, Consultant Neuroradiologist, Imperial College Healthcare NHS Trust, and Dr Gemma Dawe, Consultant Neuroradiologist, Imperial College Healthcare NHS Trust

Case 3: Positive PET study, cortical amyloid deposition

See Figure 2.22

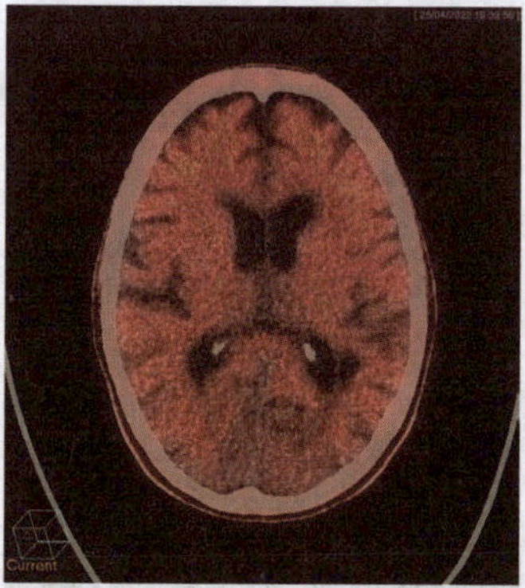

Fig. 2.22 Positive PET study, cortical amyloid deposition. Axial fused image from a florbetaben PET CT at the level of the lateral ventricles (figure 3). There is normal tracer uptake in the white matter, as seen on the negative study. However, there is abnormal tracer uptake in the grey matter, reflecting cortical amyloid deposition. This is a positive study; note the loss of grey-white matter differentiation. In normal adults without dementia, 10–20% will have positive amyloid PET scans; the value of this modality is therefore primarily in the exclusion of Alzheimer's dementia.
Reproduced courtesy of Dr Jack Garnham, Consultant Neuroradiologist, Imperial College Healthcare NHS Trust, and Dr Gemma Dawe, Consultant Neuroradiologist, Imperial College Healthcare NHS Trust

Case 4: PET control image

See Figure 2.23

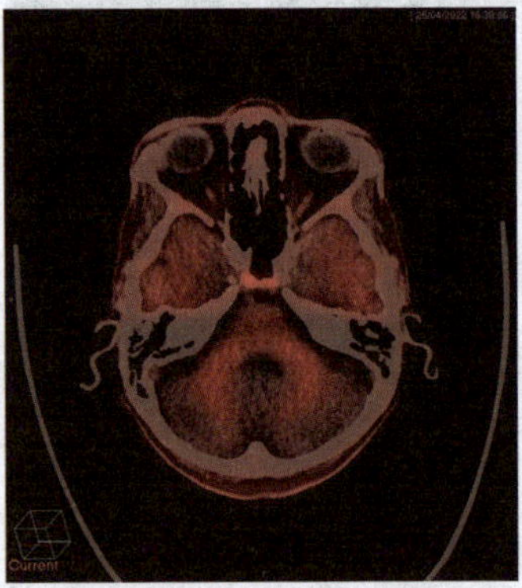

Fig. 2.23 PET control image. Axial fused image from a florbetaben PET CT at the level of the cerebellum. There is tracer uptake in the cerebellar white matter but not in the cerebellar cortex. This is seen in all studies and can be used as an internal control when assessing the supratentorial cortex.
Reproduced courtesy of Dr Jack Garnham, Consultant Neuroradiologist, Imperial College Healthcare NHS Trust, and Dr Gemma Dawe, Consultant Neuroradiologist, Imperial College Healthcare NHS Trust

Case 5: Frontotemporal dementia with 'knife blade' appearance

See Figure 2.24

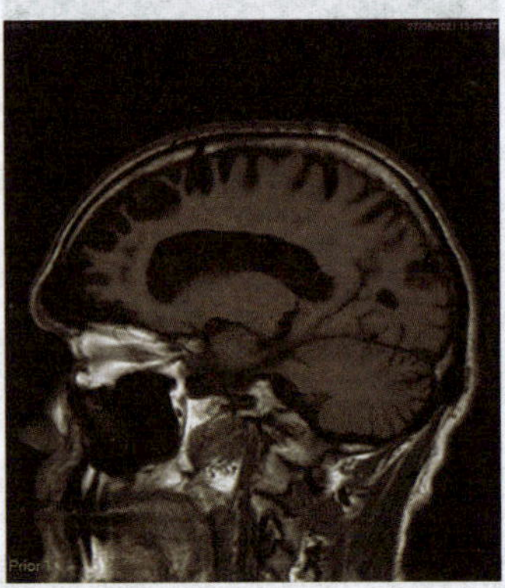

Fig. 2.24 Frontotemporal dementia with 'knife blade' appearance. Sagittal paramedian T1-weighted image of a patient with behavioural variant frontotemporal dementia. The frontal gyri are markedly thinned in comparison to the relatively normal-appearing parietal and occipital gyri; there is a pronounced anteroposterior gradient. Note the characteristic 'knife blade' appearance of the atrophic frontal gyri.
Reproduced courtesy of Dr Jack Garnham, Consultant Neuroradiologist, Imperial College Healthcare NHS Trust, and Dr Gemma Dawe, Consultant Neuroradiologist, Imperial College Healthcare NHS Trust

Case 6: Frontotemporal dementia showing thinning of the frontal gyri

See Figure 2.25

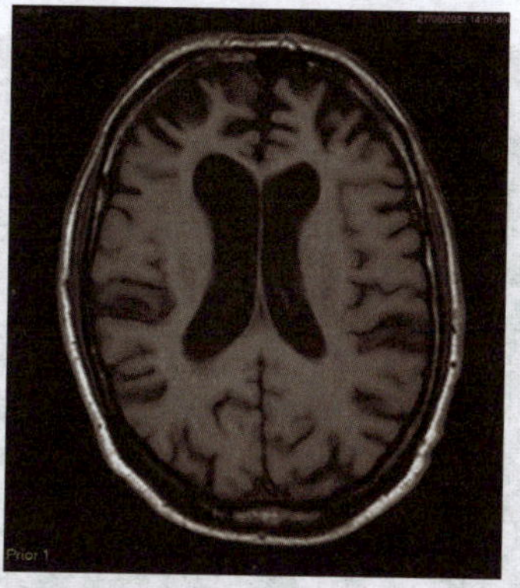

Fig. 2.25 Frontotemporal dementia showing thinning of the frontal gyri. Axial T1-weighted image of a patient with behavioural variant frontotemporal dementia at the level of the lateral ventricles. The anterior frontal gyri are thinned relative to the normal-appearing gyri elsewhere; note the anteroposterior gradient.

Reproduced courtesy of Dr Jack Garnham, Consultant Neuroradiologist, Imperial College Healthcare NHS Trust, and Dr Gemma Dawe, Consultant Neuroradiologist, Imperial College Healthcare NHS Trust

Case 7: Vascular dementia

See Figure 2.26

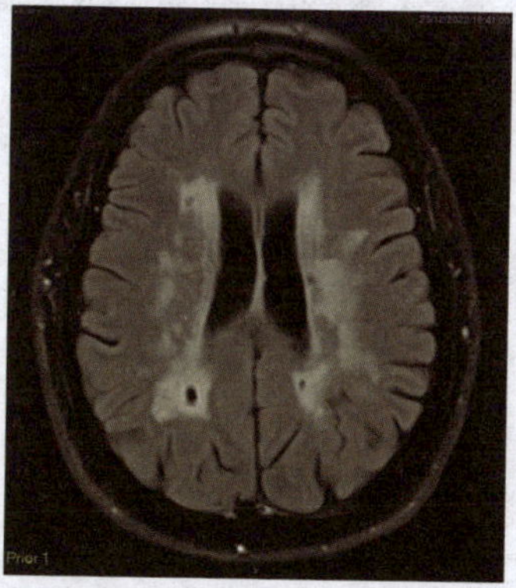

Fig. 2.26 Vascular dementia. Axial fluid attenuated inversion recovery (FLAIR) image of a patient with vascular dementia at the level of the lateral ventricles. There is patchy partially confluent hyperintensity in the periventricular and deep white matter, consistent with severe microvascular ischaemic disease. Smaller areas of low signal reflect multiple small subcortical infarcts.

Reproduced courtesy of Dr Jack Garnham, Consultant Neuroradiologist, Imperial College Healthcare NHS Trust, and Dr Gemma Dawe, Consultant Neuroradiologist, Imperial College Healthcare NHS Trust

Case 8: Normal pressure hydrocephalus

See Figure 2.27

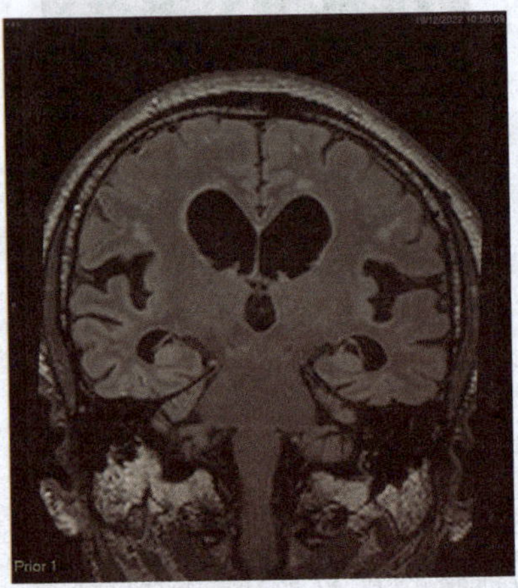

Fig. 2.27 Normal pressure hydrocephalus. Coronal FLAIR image of a patient with normal pressure hydrocephalus at the level of the posterior commissure. There is expansion of the lateral and third ventricles, asymmetrical enlargement of the Sylvian fissures, and crowding of the gyri near the vertex. The callosal angle is slightly narrowed.

Reproduced courtesy of Dr Jack Garnham, Consultant Neuroradiologist, Imperial College Healthcare NHS Trust, and Dr Gemma Dawe, Consultant Neuroradiologist, Imperial College Healthcare NHS Trust

Case 9: Progressive supranuclear palsy

See Figure 2.28

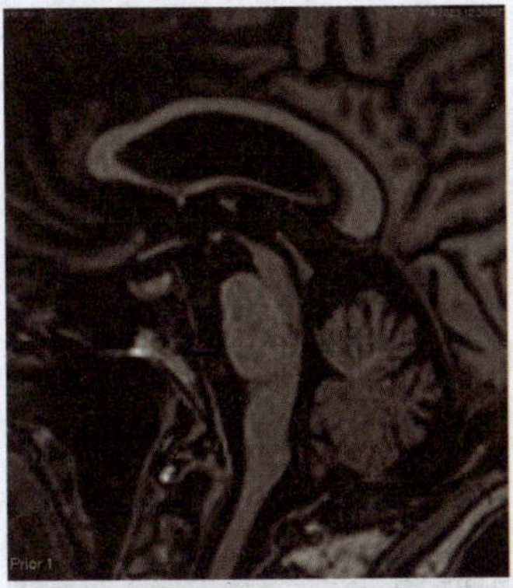

Fig. 2.28 Progressive supranuclear palsy. Midline sagittal T1-weighted image of a patient with progressive supranuclear palsy. There is midbrain volume loss with relative presentation of pontine and cerebellar volume. The normal midbrain has a convex superior border; in this patient the superior surface of the midbrain is mildly concave. The area of the midbrain on a midline sagittal image should approximate one quarter of the area of the pons; in this patient the area of the midbrain relative to the pons is reduced.

Reproduced courtesy of Dr Jack Garnham, Consultant Neuroradiologist, Imperial College Healthcare NHS Trust, and Dr Gemma Dawe, Consultant Neuroradiologist, Imperial College Healthcare NHS Trust

Case 10: Corticobasal degeneration

See Figure 2.29

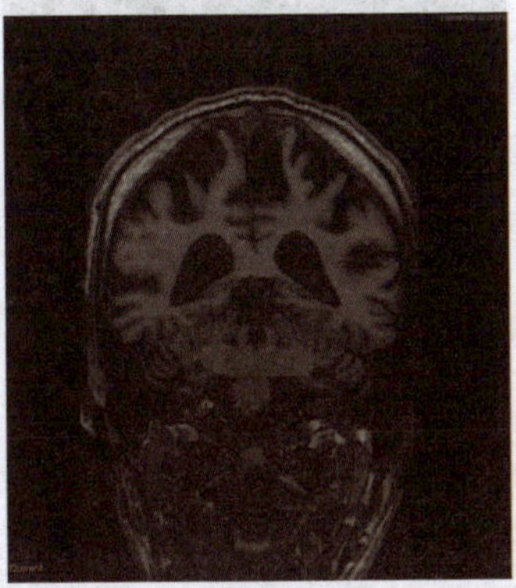

Fig. 2.29 Corticobasal degeneration. Coronal T1-weighted image of a patient with corticobasal degeneration near the level of the central sulcus. There is focal atrophy of the peri-Rolandic gyri.

Reproduced courtesy of Dr Jack Garnham, Consultant Neuroradiologist, Imperial College Healthcare NHS Trust, and Dr Gemma Dawe, Consultant Neuroradiologist, Imperial College Healthcare NHS Trust

Case 11: Corticobasal degeneration with volume loss of posterior frontal and parietal regions

See Figure 2.30

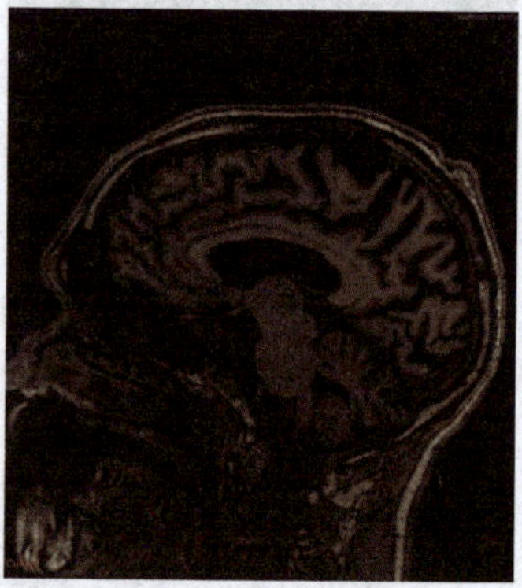

Fig. 2.30 Corticobasal degeneration with volume loss of posterior frontal and parietal regions. Sagittal paramedian T1-weighted image of a patient with corticobasal degeneration. There is volume loss affecting the posterior frontal and parietal regions, with comparative preservation of the anterior frontal gyri.
Reproduced courtesy of Dr Jack Garnham, Consultant Neuroradiologist, Imperial College Healthcare NHS Trust, and Dr Gemma Dawe, Consultant Neuroradiologist, Imperial College Healthcare NHS Trust

Case 12: Old leucotomy

See Figures 2.31a, b and 2.32

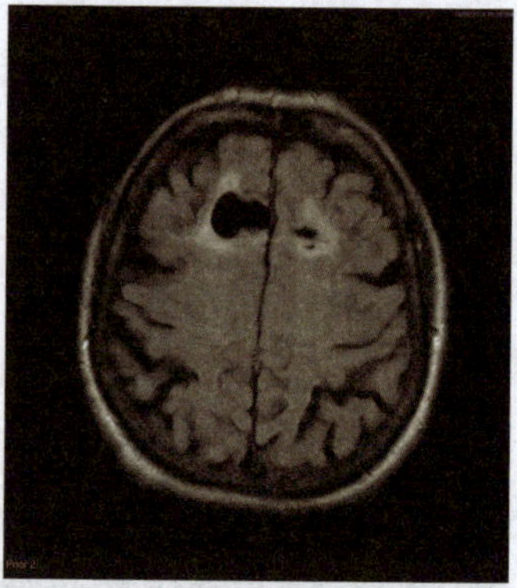

Fig. 2.31 Old leucotomy. Axial FLAIR images at the level of the centrum semiovale (a) and corona radiata (b) in a patient with a history of previous prefrontal leucotomy. There are bilateral symmetrical cavities in the frontal white matter with surrounding gliosis, characteristic of prior leucotomy.
Reproduced courtesy of Dr Jack Garnham, Consultant Neuroradiologist, Imperial College Healthcare NHS Trust, and Dr Gemma Dawe, Consultant Neuroradiologist, Imperial College Healthcare NHS Trust

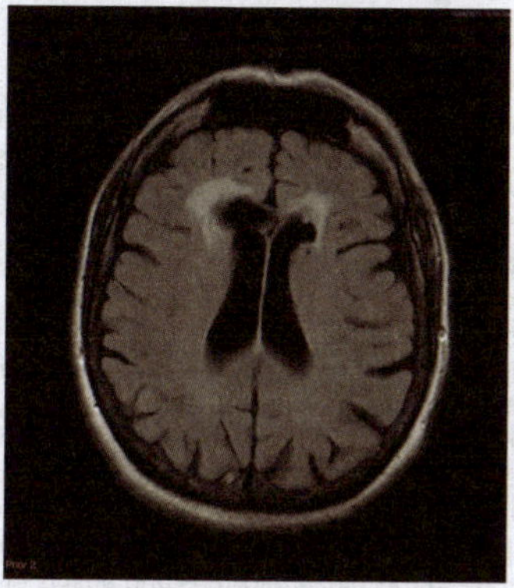

Fig. 2.31 Continued

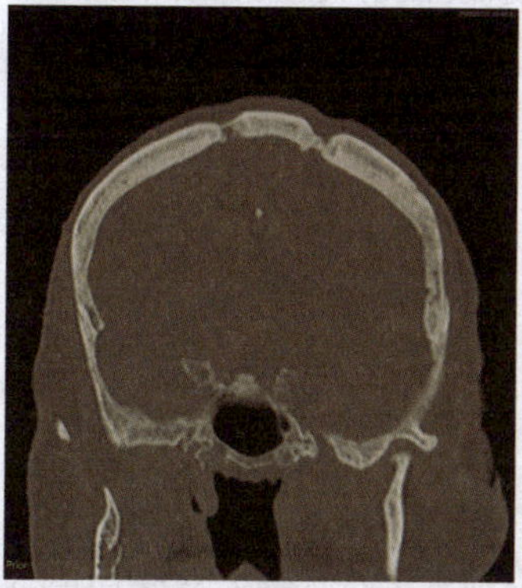

Fig. 2.32 Old leucotomy. Coronal CT image from the same patient demonstrating old bifrontal burr holes, performed as part of the leucotomy procedure.

Reproduced courtesy of Dr Jack Garnham, Consultant Neuroradiologist, Imperial College Healthcare NHS Trust, and Dr Gemma Dawe, Consultant Neuroradiologist, Imperial College Healthcare NHS Trust

Epidemiology of dementia

The global prevalence of dementia has been estimated recently as 57 million, with projections suggesting a prevalence of 153 million by 2050. The global prevalence of mild cognitive impairment is estimated to be 16% (95% confidence interval: 13–18%) for those over 50, and 17% (95% confidence interval: 13–20%) of those aged over 60[4]. Some 40–75% of these patients progress to a diagnosis of dementia with an estimated 3–4% prevalence of AD in older adults.

In clinical practice, the main aetiologies to consider are AD, vascular causes, LBD, and the FTDs. Comorbidity is common. Limbic-predominant age-related TDP-43 encephalopathy (LATE) has increasingly been recognized in patients thought to have AD but later found to have negative biomarkers. LATE tends to present more mildly, is more common in those over 90, and imaging may show hippocampal atrophy only. It can be comorbid with AD, and it is thought that this leads to a more severe presentation overall[5]. Another presentation in the 'oldest old' (80s and 90s) is primary age related tauopathy (PART), in which age-related neurofibrillary tangles are present and no amyloid pathology. These patients tend to have frontal and executive cognitive deficits and generally milder symptoms overall. In patients diagnosed with SCD, a meta analysis of longitudinal studies estimated that 27% eventually are diagnosed with MCI and 14% dementia.

Hofman et al.[1] have summarized the prevalence of dementia by age. Women tend to outnumber men from the age of 75 onwards.

Age range (years)	Prevalence rates (%)
30–59	0.1
60–64	1
65–69	1.4
70–74	4.1
75–79	5.7
80–84	13.0
85–89	21.6
90–94	32.2
95–99	34.7

Costs

It is estimated that the global cost of dementia exceeds US$1 trillion annually, corresponding to approximately US$25,000 per person. It has been well demonstrated that the presence of behavioural problems and the presence of more severe dementia increases the costs significantly. In developed countries, costs of monthly residential care range from US$4,000 to US$10,000 depending on the specific patient and country. Over 90% of patients will experience some form of BPSD, with apathy, agitation, and sleep disorders being the most common symptoms[6].

Further reading

Primary Age-Related Tauopathy (PART)[7]

Iida MA, Farrell K, Walker JM, et al. Predictors of cognitive impairment in primary age-related tauopathy: An autopsy study. Acta Neuropathol. 2021 2021/08/05;9(1):134.

Limbic-predominant age-related TDP-43 encephalopathy (LATE)

Pagnotti RMB, Pudumjee SB, Cross CL, et al. Cognitive and clinical characteristics of patients with limbic-predominant age-related TDP-43 encephalopathy. Neurology. 2023;100(19):e2027–e2035.

Subjective cognitive decline and risk of progression[8]

Jessen F, Amariglio RE, Buckley RF, et al. The characterisation of subjective cognitive decline. Lancet Neurol. 2020 Mar;19(3):271–278.

Epidemiology of BPSD in AD and FTD

Laganà V, Bruno F, Altomari N, et al. Neuropsychiatric or Behavioral and Psychological Symptoms of Dementia (BPSD): Focus on prevalence and natural history in Alzheimer's disease and frontotemporal dementia. Front Neurol. 2022;13:832199.

Reference

1. Hofman R, Rocca W, Brayne C et al. The prevalence of dementia in Europe: A collaborative study of 1980–1990 findings. Eurodem Prevalence Research Group. Int J Epidemiol. 1991 20:736–748.

Alzheimer's disease

Alois Alzheimer (1864–1915) was a psychiatrist and pathologist who combined his clinical practice with pathological examination of brains. He was a true innovator and described a number of unique microscopic stains and detailed several aspects of brain anatomy. In 1907, he published his description of a patient, Auguste D, who presented with symptoms of memory loss and paranoid delusions. At post-mortem Alzheimer found the characteristic cerebral atrophy, senile plaques, and neurofibrillary tangles seen in AD.

Signs and symptoms of AD

- Common early symptoms of AD are memory impairment and disorientation in time and place. In one-third of patients, a psychiatric problem is the presenting complaint. Memory impairment particularly affects short-term memory, and the significance of such a change is sometimes not fully appreciated by families and others (including professionals), being dismissed as a 'normal' age-related change. Changes in personality may, retrospectively, be regarded as one of the earliest signs of dementia and are well documented in the later stages. Many types of personality change are seen, including increased rigidity, increased egocentricity, impairment of regard for the feelings of others, coarsening of affect, impairment of emotional control, hilarity in inappropriate situations, diminished emotional responsiveness, sexual misdemeanour, relinquishing of hobbies, diminished initiative or growing apathy, and purposeless hyperactivity. Impairment of judgement is an important symptom that may put the patient at risk and cause concern to families.
- In addition to the changes in personality and judgement the symptoms of AD can be summarized as the 'five As': amnesia (memory loss), aphasia (language disturbance), apraxia (inability to perform motor actions), agnosia (failure to recognize persons and objects), and associated symptoms. The associated symptoms are collectively described as the behavioural and psychological symptoms of dementia (BPSD). Psychological symptoms include disorders of mood (depression and elation), disorders of thought content (delusions and paranoid ideas), and disorders of perception (hallucinations, misidentification). Behavioural disturbances include aggression, wandering, hoarding, sexual disinhibition, and eating disturbances. It is often the appearance of BPSD that caregivers find so difficult to cope with and that results in referral to specialist services.
- Several diagnostic systems exist but have broadly similar criteria. The two main umbrella systems include the Diagnostic and Statistical Manual of Mental Disorders (DSM) and the International Classification of Diseases (ICD) produced by the World Health Organization). More specialist criteria have been developed by various working groups including the National Institute on Aging and Alzheimer's Association (NIA-AA) and the International Working Group (IWG), discussed in the next section.

Criteria for diagnosis of AD

[illegible]

Cognitive profile

[illegible]

Clinical phenotypes

[illegible]

[illegible]

Criteria for diagnosis of AD

In clinical settings, a conventional process for diagnosis integrates the clinical history, assessment of function, bedside or formal cognitive testing, mental status and physical examination and neuroimaging. Taken together, it is often clear when patients are suffering from AD and this process is largely concordant with subsequent autopsy findings. More stringent criteria for research purposes would classify these patients as suffering from Alzheimer's clinical syndrome or progressive amnestic dysfunction in the absence of confirmatory biomarker evidence. Biomarkers can be helpful in clarifying the likely diagnosis if need be but have not routinely been used due to impracticality, cost, or the fact that they would not influence management. The use of blood plasma biomarkers in memory clinics may become more feasible than lumbar puncture or PET scans.

In the diagnostic process, the first step is to assess the patient's cognitive profile and rule out any relevant differential diagnoses if any deficits are found, in particular, reversible or structural causes. The next step is to assess the history and clinical phenotype present and whether this fits with a diagnosis of Alzheimer's clinical syndrome. Finally, biomarker evidence can be considered.

Cognitive profile

In general, diagnostic systems consider dementia to be present when there are significant deficits in at least two neurocognitive domains or one domain if severe deficit, and there is an impact on the person's ability to carry out their usual ADLs. In contrast, in mild cognitive impairment (MCI), one or more cognitive domains are affected but their independence isn't affected. In SCD, the patient complains of subjective impairment but formal or bedside cognitive testing is normal and the patient is independent with regard to their ADLs. Cognitively unimpaired (CU) individuals have an unremarkable assessment and the patient denies any relevant symptoms. In all cases, the differential diagnosis must be considered and other possible causes ruled out.

Clinical phenotypes

The amnestic presentation described in the previous section is most common. At earlier stages, symptoms may include short-term memory loss and the MoCA may be only mildly impaired (20–25). A variety of other atypical, non-amnestic Alzheimer's presentations exist (see Box 2.1), and often these affect younger patients and the symptoms are often misattributed to non-cortical aetiologies or misdiagnosed as functional neurological disorders. For example, posterior cortical atrophy (PCA), also known as Benson's syndrome, presents as cortical deficits in visuospatial function and praxis (see Box 2.2).

Box 2.1 Atypical Alzheimer's disease

- *Visuo-spatial:* posterior cortical atrophy (PCA).
- *Executive:* dysexecutive AD (dexAD) and behavioural variant AD (bvAD) which mimic FTD.
- *Language:* logopenic variant of primary progressive aphasia (lvPPA).
- *Motor:* corticobasal syndrome Alzheimer's disease (CBS-AD), key features include parkinsonism, myoclonus, and alien limb phenomena.

Box 2.2 Posterior cortical atrophy (Benson's syndrome)

Differential diagnosis: The differential includes LBD, vascular cognitive impairment, corticobasal syndrome, and prion disease. *Clinical features:* patients are younger than typical AD. Patients may experience symptoms of apraxia and difficulty in navigating the world around them due to cortical visual deficits:

- Visuospatial deficits including neglect
- Prosopagnosia
- Balint's syndrome: simultagnosia, optic ataxia, ocular motor apraxia
- Gerstmann's syndrome: agraphia, finger agnosia, acalculia, left-right disorientation
- Apraxia

Neuropsychological tests: a Navon figure (Fig. 2.33), an image made of smaller images, e.g. a letter T made up of smaller letter Ps can be used to test for neglect and simultagnosia. Patients will not be able to recognize the larger figure. Visuospatial tasks will be difficult, including cube and clock drawing. *Imaging* may show occipito-parietal deficits. *Management* includes consideration of AChEIs or memantine.

PPPPPPPPPPPPPPPPPPPPPPPPPP

PPPPPPPPPPPPPPPPPPPPPPPPPP

PPPPPP

PPPPPP

PPPPPP

PPPPPP

PPPPPP

PPPPPP

Fig. 2.33 Navon figure of the letter T made up of Ps.

Biomarkers

In clinical practice, structural neuroimaging is routinely performed whereas lumbar punctures and PET scans are usually not unless there is diagnostic uncertainty. Blood-based plasma biomarkers may be more convenient for routine practice, but their use and interpretation need to be thoughtfully considered when counselling patients.

In most diagnostic systems, dementia or MCI must be present for a diagnosis of AD. However, 2024 NIA-AA criteria, which are purely biological, allow for a diagnosis of AD if biomarkers are positive even in cognitively unimpaired (CU) individuals[9]. In contrast, IWG criteria consider biomarker positive, CU individuals to be 'at risk of progression' because of the uncertainty of what these positive tests are actually predicting[10]. See Dubois et al. (2021) for an in-depth discussion.

Biomarkers can be divided into amyloid, tau, and non-specific markers. Amyloid tests include low CSF Aβ 42 (or Aβ 42/40 ratio) or a positive amyloid PET scan. Tau tests include positive tau PET, raised phosphorylated tau in the CSF, or blood plasma tests for hyperphosphorylated tau (e.g. p-tau 181, p-tau 217). Non-specific markers include MRI atrophy and FDG-PET changes. Emerging blood tests include neurofilament light chain (NfL), suggestive of axonal damage, and astrocytic glial fibrillary acidic protein (GFAP), suggestive of inflammation.

Further reading

An excellent textbook with an in-depth guide to diagnosis[11]

Budson A, Solomon, P (2023). Chapters 1–4. In: *Memory loss, Alzheimer's disease and dementia.* Philadelphia, PA: Elsevier.

Vascular cognitive impairment and vascular dementia

The concept of cognitive deficits linked to vascular injury has broadened to include [illegible] vascular cognitive impairment (VCI).

Differentiation between AD and vascular dementia (VaD) [illegible]

Diagnostic criteria

VCI is divided into mild VCI [illegible] Major VCI or VaD [illegible]

- [illegible] within 6 months of stroke.
- Subcortical ischaemic vascular dementia: small vessel disease, mainly [illegible]
- Multi-infarct dementia [illegible]

Presentation

Classic cases of VaD [illegible] cerebrovascular accident. The course is [illegible] stepwise progression [illegible]

Examination

Neurological examination

- Focal neurological signs [illegible] with stroke.
- [illegible]
- History [illegible]
- [illegible]

Vascular cognitive impairment and vascular dementia

The concept of cognitive deficits linked to vascular injury has broadened to include milder cognitive impairment under the umbrella of 'vascular cognitive impairment' (VCI).

Differentiation between AD and vascular dementia (VaD) in elderly people can be difficult during life and an accurate diagnosis often depends on a reliable informant supplying a collateral history.

Diagnostic criteria

VCI is divided into mild VCI and major VCI, which corresponds to VaD. Major VCI or VaD requires that dementia is diagnosed in terms of cognitive domain and functional impairment. Major VCI or VaD is then further subdivided into four diagnostic categories according to the Vascular Impairment of Cognition Classification Consensus Study (VICCCS) criteria(12,13). Structural MRI is the recommended imaging modality:

- Post-stroke dementia (PSD): cognitive impairment within 6 months of stroke.
- Subcortical ischaemic vascular dementia: small vessel disease, mainly subcortical lesions. This includes Binswanger's disease (subcortical arteriosclerotic encephalopathy) and the lacunar state.
- Multi-infarct (cortical) dementia: multiple, large cortical infarcts are present.
- Mixed dementia: mixed diagnostic picture, e.g. VCI-AD, VCI-DLB.

Presentation

Classical onset of VaD is sudden and follows a clearly definable cerebrovascular accident. The course is usually described as a stepwise progression with episodes of clouding of consciousness and subsequently a fluctuating level of cognitive impairment. Apoplectiform features punctuate the progress of the disorder and are due to episodes of infarction. Commonly they consist of abrupt episodes of hemiparesis, sensory change, dysphasia, or visual disturbances. At first they can be transient and followed by gradual restitution of function, but later on permanent neurological deficits appear. When the onset is more gradual, non-cognitive changes are said to pre-date the impairments of memory and intellect. There is greater mood lability and a greater tendency toward depression and anxiety than is commonly seen in AD. Very occasionally lacunar infarcts can be associated with gradual mental deterioration without focal signs. Other early features include somatic symptoms such as headache, dizziness, tinnitus, and syncope, which may be the main complaints for some time prior to diagnosis.

Examination

Physical examination

- Focal neurological signs (such as hemiparesis, lower facial weakness, Babinski sign, sensory deficit, hemianopia, and dysarthria consistent with stroke).
- Early presence of a gait disturbance (small-step gait or *marche a petit pas*, or magnetic apraxic–ataxic or parkinsonian gait).
- History of unsteadiness and frequent, unprovoked falls.
- Early urinary frequency, urgency, and other urinary symptoms not explained by urinary disease.

Mental State Examination

- Personality and mood changes, abulia, depression, emotional incontinence, and other subcortical deficits including psychomotor retardation and abnormal executive function.
- Pseudolbulbar affect (PBA): pathological laughing and crying characterized by incongruent, involuntary outbursts.

Investigations

Neuropsychological testing

The patchy nature of the psychological deficits in contrast to the global impairment of AD is said to distinguish between the two types of dementia with relative preservation of personality and insight in VCI.

Imaging

MRI can demonstrate large cortical infarcts or subcortical ischaemia. The Fazekas score can quantify white matter hyperintensities. Scoring ranges from 0 to 3; 0, no or a single punctate WMH lesion; 1, indicating multiple punctate lesions; 2, bridging of lesions; 3, large, confluent WMH lesions.

Differential diagnosis

In general, the clinical features that have been found to be most accurate in differentiating vascular and Alzheimer-type dementia include neurological signs and symptoms, a history of strokes, hypertension, and abrupt onset. The key features that distinguish between AD and VaD were described by Hachinski et al.[1] and made into a checklist from which a score (the Hachinski score) is derived. The original score was based on features of VaD in a textbook of psychiatry and studies of the cerebral blood flow in patients with dementia. The initial study group were relatively young and more mildly affected by their illness than are patients seen in most old age psychiatry services. A bimodal distribution of scores was found and suggested that patients with a score below 4 had a dementia of the Alzheimer's type and those having a score of 7 or above a VaD. Patients scoring between 4 and 7 were thought to have a mixed picture. These key features are shown in Box 2.3.

Box 2.3 The Hachinski ischaemic score elements

- Abrupt onset
- Stepwise progression
- Fluctuating course
- Normal confusion
- Relative presentation of personality
- Depression
- Somatic complaints
- Emotional incontinence
- History of hypertension
- History of strokes
- Evidence of associated atherosclerosis
- Focal neurological symptoms
- Focal neurological signs

Source: data from Hachinski VC, Iliff LD, Zilhka E et al. Cerebral blood flow in dementia. Arch Neurol. 1975;32(9):632–637[4]

However, the validity of using the Hachinski score to differentiate between VaDs and other types of dementias has been questioned. The Hachinski score has been criticized as not being sufficiently sensitive. Moreover, higher scores on the Hachinski do not reliably make a diagnosis of VaD more likely and the checklist does not take into account results from neuroradiological examinations. Infarctions are common in older people, including those with AD, and thus a mixed picture is common.

Further reading

The VICCCS Criteria

Skrobot OA, Black SE, Chen C, et al. Progress toward standardized diagnosis of vascular cognitive impairment: Guidelines from the Vascular Impairment of Cognition Classification Consensus Study. Alzheimers Dement. 2018 Mar;14(3):280–292.

Reference

1. Hachinski VC, Iliff LD, Zilhka E et al. Cerebral blood flow in dementia. Arch Neurol. 1975;32(9):632–637.

Dementia with Lewy bodies

Dementia with Lewy bodies (DLB) is characterized by a fluctuating course with distressing psychotic symptoms and marked behavioural disturbance interspersed with periods of lucidity where the degree of cognitive impairment seems relatively minor in relation to the severity of the behavioural disturbance. The psychiatric symptoms may be the presenting feature or may appear in the context of long-standing Parkinson's disease. Sleep disturbance, autonomic lability, and marked sensitivity to neuroleptic drugs are also characteristic of the illness. At times it can be difficult to differentiate between VCI and DLB and as with AD and VCI a mixed picture is not uncommon.

History

The core features of DLB are *fluctuation of cognition* with pronounced variations in attention and alertness; spontaneous motor features of *parkinsonism*; recurrent *visual hallucinations* which are typically well formed and detailed and *REM sleep behaviour disorder* (RBD). At least 2 of these 4 symptoms are required for a probable diagnosis, with or without biomarker evidence (see Box 2.4 for full diagnostic criteria). Features supportive of the diagnosis are autonomic dysfunctions, repeated falls, syncope, hyposmia, transient loss of consciousness, neuroleptic sensitivity, systematized delusions, and hallucinations (other than visual).

Box 2.4 Revised criteria for the clinical diagnosis of dementia with Lewy bodies (DLB)

Essential for a diagnosis of DLB is dementia, defined as a progressive cognitive decline of sufficient magnitude to interfere with normal social or occupational functions, or with usual daily activities. Prominent or persistent memory impairment may not necessarily occur in the early stages but is usually evident with progression. Deficits on tests of attention, executive function, and visuoperceptual ability may be especially prominent and occur early.

Core clinical features (the first 3 typically occur early and may persist throughout the course)

- Fluctuating cognition with pronounced variations in attention and alertness.
- Recurrent visual hallucinations that are typically well formed and detailed.
- REM sleep behaviour disorder, which may precede cognitive decline.
- One or more spontaneous cardinal features of parkinsonism: these are bradykinesia (defined as slowness of movement and decrement in amplitude or speed), rest tremor, or rigidity.

Supportive clinical features

- Severe sensitivity to antipsychotic agents.
- Postural instability.
- Repeated falls.
- Syncope or other transient episodes of unresponsiveness.
- Severe autonomic dysfunction, e.g. constipation, orthostatic hypotension, urinary incontinence.

Box 2.4 *(Contd.)*

- Hypersomnia.
- Hyposmia.
- Hallucinations in other modalities.
- Systematized delusions.
- Apathy, anxiety, and depression.

Indicative biomarkers

Reduced dopamine transporter uptake in basal ganglia demonstrated by SPECT or PET. Abnormal (low uptake) 123I-MIBG myocardial scintigraphy.

Polysomnographic confirmation of REM sleep without atonia.

Supportive biomarkers

Relative preservation of medial temporal lobe structures on CT/MRI scan.

Generalized low uptake on SPECT/PET perfusion/metabolism scan with reduced occipital activity with or without the cingulate island sign on FDG-PET imaging.

Prominent posterior slow-wave activity on EEG with periodic fluctuations in the pre-alpha/ theta range.

Probable DLB can be diagnosed if:

a. Two or more core clinical features of DLB are present, with or without the presence of indicative biomarkers, or
b. Only one core clinical feature is present, but with one or more indicative biomarkers.
Probable DLB should not be diagnosed on the basis of biomarkers alone.

Possible DLB can be diagnosed if:

a. Only one core clinical feature of DLB is present, with no indicative biomarker evidence; or
b. One or more indicative biomarkers is present but there are no core clinical features.

DLB is less likely:

a. In the presence of any other physical illness or brain disorder including cerebrovascular disease, sufficient to account in part or in total for the clinical picture, although these do not exclude a DLB diagnosis and may serve to indicate mixed or multiple pathologies contributing to the clinical presentation; or
b. If parkinsonian features are the only core clinical feature and appear for the first time at a stage of severe dementia.

Notes

DLB should be diagnosed when dementia occurs before or concurrently with parkinsonism.

The term 'Parkinson disease dementia' (PDD) should be used to describe dementia that occurs in the context of well-established Parkinson disease.

In a practice setting the term that is most appropriate to the clinical situation should be used and generic terms such as 'Lewy body disease' are often helpful.

(Continued)

Box 2.4 *(Contd.)*

In research studies in which distinction needs to be made between DLB and PDD, the existing 1-year rule between the onset of dementia and parkinsonism continues to be recommended.

Examination

Physical examination

- Neurological examination: parkinsonism suggested by the triad of tremor, rigidity, and bradykinesia. Tremor is 'pill rolling' and worse at rest. The patient's face may be mask like and hypomimetic. Shuffling, festinant gait. Tone increased on examination. Lack of habituation to blinking elicited by glabellar tapping (glabellar tap reflex) is known as Myerson's sign.

Mental State Examination

- Psychotic symptoms can be quite vivid in nature. Visual hallucinations (VH) often revolve around animals, children, or miniaturized versions of people. Diffusion tensor imaging (DTI) suggests that, in comparison to DLB without VH, this is due to disruption of the inferior longitudinal fasciculus which forms part of a circuit with the occipital lobe visual association cortex and the amygdala (visuo-amygdaloid pathway)[14,15].
- Other hallucinations include the feeling that someone, or a group of people are present ('presence hallucinations') and that something or someone is moving in the periphery of their vision ('passage hallucinations').
- Delusions may encompass themes such as theft, infidelity or the television coming to life. Delusional misidentification has been reported, e.g. Capgras syndrome where familiar persons have been replaced by an identical looking imposter.
- Hypnagogic (falling asleep) and hypnopompic (awakening) hallucinations may be present, especially in the presence of RBD.

Investigations

Neuropsychological testing

- Deficits on visuospatial ability, tests of attention, and frontal/subcortical skills may be prominent and memory impairment may not necessarily occur in the early stages but may be evident with progression.

Imaging

- DaT scan: reduced dopamine transporter uptake in basal ganglia by SPECT or PET.
- Abnormal (low-uptake) 123 iodine-MIBG myocardial scintigraphy.
- MRI: relative preservation of medial temporal lobe structures on CT/MRI scan.
- Generalized low uptake on SPECT/PET perfusion/metabolism scan with reduced occipital activity ± cingulate island sign on FDG-PET imaging.

Polysomnography

- Polysomnographic confirmation of REM sleep without atonia.

See section *Drug treatment in non-Alzheimer's dementia for management.*

Further reading

Simple pen and paper tasks to distinguish parkinsonian from essential tremor[16]

Alty J, Cosgrove J, Thorpe D, et al. How to use pen and paper tasks to aid tremor diagnosis in the clinic. Pract Neurol. 2017;17(6):456–463.

Dementias in the context of other neurological disorders

Sometimes neurocognitive deficits at the severity of dementia are part of a constellation of other symptoms in the context of other neurological disorders. Cognitive deficit or neuropsychiatric symptoms are often the presenting complaint rather than the more familiar motor manifestations. General diagnostic categories to think about are parkinsonian disorders, choreiform disorders, and ataxic disorders.

Parkinson's plus syndromes

There are several 'Parkinson's plus' syndromes, which can either present with cognitive problems or progress to dementia with neuropsychiatric symptoms. Parkinsonism can also develop due to vascular disease, which tends to be symmetrical without tremor ('vascular parkinsonism', see *vascular cognitive impairment* section).

Progressive supranuclear palsy (PSP)

Also known as Steele–Richardson–Olszewski syndrome, this is an atypical parkinsonian disorder with supranuclear gaze palsy which presents in patients over age 65, equally in males and females. The underlying pathology is a tauopathy. *Clinical features:* the core clinical features of PSP are a tetrad of akinesia (parkinsonian features), oculomotor dysfunction (in particular, vertical gaze palsy), postural instability, and neurocognitive deficits[17]. Regarding cognition, deficits are mainly frontal and the 6-question frontal assessment battery (FAB) may be a useful test. There may be progressive apraxia of speech and non-fluent aphasia. *Investigations:* MRI may show characteristic signs indicative of midbrain atrophy, including the 'hummingbird', 'mickey mouse', and 'morning glory' signs. *Management:* dopaminergic medications are less useful but often trialled. There is less risk of impulse control disorders (ICDs) than in PD. Cholinesterase inhibitors have little evidence of efficacy. Citalopram, trazodone, mirtazapine, and rTMS have been used to treat depressive symptoms in PSP[18].

Corticobasal syndrome

Corticobasal syndrome (CBS) commonly presents with cognitive symptoms. CBS refers to the clinical syndrome of motor symptoms (atypical parkinsonism, dystonia, apraxia, myoclonus), 'alien limb phenomena', and cortical sensory symptoms. Simultagnosia, graphaesthesia (i.e. inability to recognize a letter drawn onto the palm), and astereognosis (i.e. cannot recognize a pen by feeling it) may be present. Alien limb phenomena are described by patients feeling as if their arm or hand is not their own, or that it is missing, or being controlled by something else. However, this should be distinguished from passivity symptoms in the psychotic disorders.

Dementia is the most common presentation, and in contrast to AD, there is less memory impairment and more parietal lobe deficits[19]. Neuropsychiatric symptoms include depression, irritability, apathy, compulsive behaviours, and sometimes FTD-like disinhibition.

The underlying pathology is diverse, and only about half have been found to have corticobasal degeneration (CBD) at postmortem, a 4-repeat tauopathy with astrocytic plaques-[20]. The remaining cases consist of PSP,

AD, frontotemporal lobar degeneration (FTLD), DLB, and others. Myoclonus and posterior cortical signs (e.g. dyscalculia) are more predictive of CBD. Asymmetrical motor or sensory signs, hyperreflexia, and gait impairment have been found to help distinguish early CBD from AD[21].

Management includes controlling motor symptoms and standard antidepressant therapy. There is a dearth of any studies of cholinesterase inhibitors or memantine.

Multiple system atrophy

Multiple system atrophy (MSA) is a rare alpha-synucleinopathy affecting oligodendrocytes. Symptoms can include parkinsonism, cerebellar signs, and autonomic dysfunction depending on the subtype. In MSA, mild cognitive impairment has been found in up to approximately 40% of patients, with 11% diagnosed with dementia, usually in the later stages[22]. Patients may have more frontal deficits on cognitive testing.

Choreiform disorders

Huntington's disease

Neuropsychiatric symptoms, particularly depression, commonly occur before motor symptoms and there is an increased suicide risk. Other symptoms include frontal disinhibition, psychosis in up to 10%, and obsessive–compulsive disorder (OCD) in up to roughly half of patients. Compared to AD, executive dysfunction and social cognitive deficits are more prominent and memory loss occurs later. Patients suffering from Huntington's disease (HD) may have more difficulty in tasks such as the Wisconsin card sorting test and sequencing tasks.

A small study of donepezil did not show any effect on cognition or motor symptoms in HD[23]. Selective serotonin reuptake inhibitors (SSRIs) can be used to manage mood and OCD symptoms. Antipsychotics such as olanzapine may be helpful for both BPSD and chorea. Brief prescriptions of low-dose benzodiazepines (e.g. lorazepam 0.5 mg) are often used in crisis or difficult to manage agitation. If sleep is disordered, sedating antidepressants (e.g. mirtazapine) or atypical antipsychotics could be considered; melatonin has also been utilized[24]. For apathy, suggestions include serotonin and norepinephrine reuptake inhibitors (SNRIs) (e.g. venlafaxine, duloxetine), stimulants, or atomoxetine (see *BPSD* section).

Ataxic disorders

Cerebellar cognitive affective syndrome (Schmahmann's syndrome)

Whilst the cerebellum was previously thought to only be associated with motor and vestibular functions, it also plays a role in cognition and affect. Just as damage to the anterior cerebellum can cause dysmetria of motor control, damage to the posterior cerebellum can cause dysmetria of thought[25]. The group of symptoms which occur when the cognitive cerebellum is affected is called the cerebellar cognitive affective syndrome (CCAS) and the CCAS Scale can be used as a screener[25]. From a neuropsychiatric perspective, the picture appears to mimic a frontal-dysexecutive syndrome but it has particular features. Patients may experience disinhibition and apathy rather than agitation or aggression. Other features may include flattened affect, difficulties in emotional control, social cognitive deficits, psychotic symptoms, and OCD symptomatology. Mutism may be present (cerebellar mutism)[26]. Regarding memory, deficits are primarily in working memory and in executive control of memory (i.e. speed of retrieval) rather than memory storage. Other deficits are linguistic (dysprosodia, anomia, agrammatism) and visuospatial, with difficulties in tasks using 3-dimensional rather than 2-dimensional images. The underlying aetiology is diverse. There is case report evidence for donepezil in managing CCAS[27].

Further reading:

PSP diagnostic checklist

Höglinger GU, Respondek G, Stamelou M, et al. Clinical diagnosis of progressive supranuclear palsy: The movement disorder society criteria. Mov Disord. 2017 Jun;32(6):853–864.

The clinico-pathological method applied to corticobasal syndrome

Shir D, Pham NTT, Botha H, et al. Clinicoradiologic and neuropathologic evaluation of corticobasal syndrome. Neurology. 2023 Jul 18;101(3):e289–e299.

Cerebellar dementia[28]

Toniolo S, Pisotta I, Manto M. Editorial: The role of the cerebellum in dementia and neurodegenerative diseases. Front Neurosci. 2023;17:1229624.

CCAS-Scale

Hoche F, Guell X, Vangel MG, et al. The cerebellar cognitive affective/Schmahmann syndrome scale. Brain. 2018 Jan 1;141(1):248–270.

Donepezil for Cerebellar Cognitive Affective Syndrome

Nishida Y, Hizume M, Fumimura Y, et al. Cerebellar cognitive affective syndrome improved by donepezil. Intern Med. 2019 Apr 1;58(7):1003–1006.

Neuropathology in AD

Neuropathological methods

In disease states, the cells of the nervous system will respond with 'pathologic reactions' which can be classified and identified. In pathology, these are identified with both macroscopic examination of the brain and microscopic examination of neural tissue. In microscopic analysis, stains are used to demonstrate morphology of the tissue and thus help to identify any pathologic reactions. Two key methods in microscopic analysis are the use of tinctorial stains, such as haematoxylin and eosin (H&E), which can show key structural features, and secondly, immunohistochemical methods, which enable visualization of specific antigens. This enables molecular phenotyping and informs basic scientific investigations into the underlying neurobiology.

The underlying pathology crucially informs the use of biological markers ('biomarkers') of disease, which are quantifiable medical surrogates for the underlying pathology. The exact nature of the relationship between surrogate and pathology lies behind current controversies around positive AD biomarkers in cognitively unimpaired individuals (see *Alzheimer's disease* section for discussion). Looking to oncology for analogy, the use of surrogates as endpoints in clinical trials has been pragmatic but introduces problems of interpretation.

Macroscopic findings

The most obvious finding on the naked eye examination is generalized atrophy of the cerebral hemispheres but in particular the medial temporal lobes and hippocampal regions (Fig. 2.34).

Microscopic findings

Throughout the microscopic pathology the most distinctive and widespread are senile (neuritic) plaques and neurofibrillary tangles (Fig. 2.35). Plaques are best seen with silver stain or immunocytochemistry using antibodies to β-amyloid peptide. These are extracellular plaques and consist of a dense core surrounded by less dense material. These neuritic plaques may well be the successor of diffuse plaques which consist of deposits of fibrillary material without any evidence of a central core of amyloid. Neurofibrillary tangles (NFTs) are abnormal structures inside neurones and are well seen with silver stains or using immunocytochemical stains of antibodies against their principal component, hyperphosphorylated tau. They are smaller than

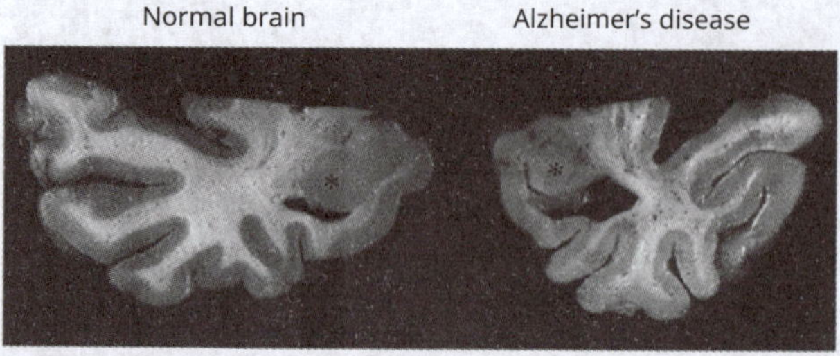

Fig. 2.34 Normal brain compared with Alzheimer brain showing widespread atrophy.
Reproduced from Dawdarn D, Allen S (eds), *Neurobiology of Alzheimer's disease* 3rd edn. Oxford: Oxford University Press.

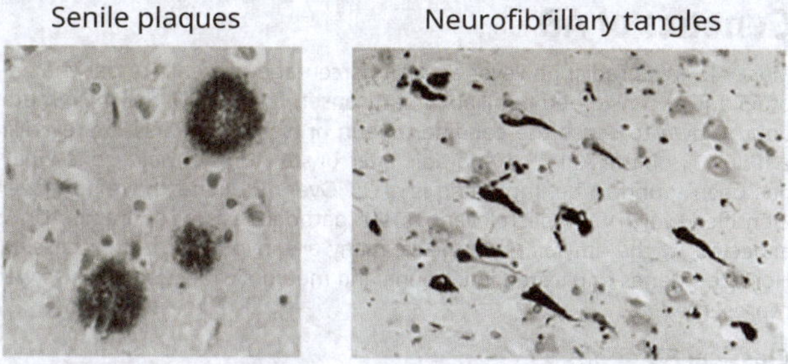

Fig. 2.35 Senile plaques and NFTs.
Reproduced from Dawdarn D, Allen S (eds), *Neurobiology of Alzheimer's disease* 3rd edn. Oxford: Oxford University Press.

plaques and most contain a nuclear core although some tangles are clearly extracellular and appear to be the result of neuronal death (a 'ghost' tangle). Braak staging refers to a method of assessing the characteristic spread of neurofibrillary pathology starting in the transentorhinal region, to limbic regions and then more diffusely.

The main component of the plaque is a peptide (amyloid-β, Aβ) which is derived from the amyloid precursor protein (APP). The Aβ peptide, popularly known as amyloid, is a 40–42 amino acid product which is formed from the abnormal metabolism of the much larger (120 amino acid) APP. This breakdown appears to be caused by secretase enzymes; single genes for these secretase enzymes may by mutation be sufficient to cause familial cases of early-onset AD. Though rare, such cases have allowed a joined-up understanding of the cascade of events which allows metabolic perturbations to result in the clinical expression of commonly found AD. The postulated series of pathological events caused by the various forms of Aβ is sometimes referred to as the 'amyloid cascade' hypothesis.

Identification of pathological brain network architecture

In addition to traditional pathological methods, there is an increasing trend of characterizing pathology at the level of brain networks *in vivo* using functional network biomarkers. Functional MRI (fMRI) can identify spatially distinct brain regions which have temporally correlated levels of activity, which is also called 'functional connectivity' (i.e. two neural regions far apart could be active at the same time). This is based on the blood-oxygen level dependent level (BOLD) signal, a measure of blood flow and hence a surrogate marker of neuronal activity. Using this method, several key brain networks have been identified, including the default mode network (DMN) which is active when subjects appear to be simply lying in a scanner and not engaged in any task at all ('resting state' fMRI). The 'network degeneration hypothesis' can help to explain why the same pathological reaction can produce different symptoms by affecting different brain networks, and how distinct aetiological mechanisms can affect the same brain network and appear similar clinically. Importantly, it can also identify therapeutic targets.

In both AD and MCI, alterations have been observed in the default mode, salience, and limbic networks. In DLB, motor networks are more likely to be affected than in AD. As expected, frontal regions are disrupted in FTD but also key limbic hubs and networks involving the basal ganglia.

Genetics of AD

Most AD is sporadic, however a small percentage presents under the age of 65 and is considered familial. In early-onset, familial AD, the main mutations known to cause the condition are in presenilin 1 (PSEN1), presenilin 2 (PSEN2), or the APP. For sporadic later onset AD, the main gene which has been found to be implicated is *APOE*. Over 200 genes have now been identified which may be relevant to the pathogenesis of sporadic AD. As expected by the amyloid hypothesis, many are involved in Aβ processing. However, genes implicated in immune and metabolic function are also well represented.

Classical AD genes

- **Amyloid precursor protein:** The main component of the plaque is the peptide Aβ which is derived from APP. A number of mutations were found in the gene encoding for APP in the early to mid-1980s, the first familial gene to be found in AD, in particular in chromosome 21 which fitted neatly with the observation that Down's syndrome (caused by trisomy 21 in the majority of people) is often associated with AD. Several more *APP* mutations have been described.
- **Presenilin mutations:** Another group of genetic abnormalities are the presenilin mutations. These are transmembrane proteins and the genes *PS1* (linked to chromosome 14) and *PS2* (linked to chromosome 1) have been described, the former appearing to be a dominant, early-onset familial chain for AD.
- **Apolipoprotein E (*APOE*)** is linked to chromosome 19 and is a polymorphic gene that exists in three alleles—*e2*, *e3*, and *e4*—containing different amino acids. *e3* is the most common allele followed by *e4* and *e2*. Any individual has any two of these three resulting in either being homozygous (*e2/e2*, *e3/e3*, *e4/e4*) or heterozygous (*e2/e3*, *e2/e4*, *e3/e4*) in phenotype. The presence of either one or two of the *e4* alleles has been associated with the development of cardiovascular disease and a number of studies have documented the greatly increased risk of AD in people with one or two *e4* alleles. APOE is a lipid transport molecule and is a liver-synthesized very low density lipoprotein. Figures vary between studies, but in people with familial AD compared with controls, 20% and 2%, respectively had *e4/e4*, 57% and 21%, respectively, had *e3/e4* and 20% and 57%, respectively, had *e3/e3*. There is some evidence to show that *e4* may be specifically related to the formation of NFTs and amyloid. The APOE *e4* allele increases risk of developing AD and the disease comes on at an earlier age than expected.
- There is some evidence that e4 carriers have superior visual working memory[29]. This may be an example of the antagonistic pleiotropy theory of ageing[30]. Pleiotropy refers to the multiple effects of a gene or allele. This theory posits that alleles which are favourable early on in life often are deleterious later on in life. This trade-off may be because natural selection's effects are lessened post reproduction and therefore these alleles can accumulate in the genome. Conversely, longevity alleles often are found to reduce survival or reproductive success in earlier life.

Can relatives have tests to show their risks of AD?

This question is sometimes asked by relatives but is also often clearly in the back of their minds. In practice, in those rare families in whom there is a clear autosomal dominant pedigree with early onset (fifth or sixth decade), then genetic testing may reveal a characteristic mutation which makes development of the condition inevitable. Clinical geneticists often handle the implications of testing with such families. Understandably, some might choose not to know. Much more common is being asked by the middle-aged children of older people with dementia whether there is any way of checking their risk. *APOE e4* genotyping is the main candidate and it can be obtained commercially now by patients themselves. However, it is not used in routine clinical practice as the rate of false positives and false negatives is high and interpretation of any results must be done with care. It is estimated *APOE e4* alleles increases the risk of AD by a ratio of 3:8[31].

Neurochemistry in AD

Mediating the cognitive and neuropsychiatric symptoms observed in AD are alterations in neurotransmitter and synaptic function. The main neurotransmitters affected earlier on in the course of disease are cholinergic, glutamatergic, and monoaminergic. However, as the disease progresses from hippocampal to cortical regions, the other principal neurotransmitter systems in the brain become dysregulated too. Although a short summary of the key neurotransmitters is presented below, synergism and complex interactions between neurotransmitters is the rule rather than the exception.

Acetylcholine

The concept of cholinergic dysfunction being central to AD is known as the cholinergic hypothesis[23][32]. This neurotransmitter is involved in vital cholinergic pathways projecting from the basal forebrain and brainstem to the cerebral cortex. Functionally, these circuits are involved in normal perception, learning, attention, cognition, and judgement. Early loss of cholinergic neurons in the basal forebrain nucleus basalis of Meynert has been established for decades as part of the AD disease process. Substantial loss of the enzyme choline acetyltransferase, required for synthesis of acetylcholine, has been demonstrated pre- and post-mortem, while loss of nicotinic receptors in the brains of AD patients has been reported. Importantly, the magnitude of cholinergic dysfunction is proportional to both neuropathological changes in AD and to the degree of cognitive impairment. Finally, the acetylcholinesterase inhibitors (AChEIs) are the longest-established evidence based treatments for AD and act by restoring cholinergic function.

Glutamate

Glutamate is an excitatory neurotransmitter which acts diffusely, including through the N-methyl-D-aspartate (NMDA) receptor. Glutamatergic neurons degenerate early in AD. Neuronal cell death in many conditions is mediated by the effects of glutamate at the NMDA receptor, while the NMDA antagonist memantine is licensed for treatment in later dementia, especially in AD.

Noradrenaline

Noradrenergic neurons project to the amygdala, thalamus, and cortex from brainstem nuclei. The noradrenergic system is important for alertness, memory, and attention. Though damage to noradrenergic nuclei has been shown in AD (especially to the locus coeruleus early on), its clinical significance is unclear. A meta-analysis of the effects of a range of noradrenergic medications in AD suggest that it is plausible they could improve general cognition as opposed to neuropsychiatric symptoms[33]. Interestingly, these medications are standard treatments for ADHD, such as methylphenidate, atomoxetine, and guanfacine. Another approach to addressing noradrenergic deficit is via direct stimulation of the locus coeruleus using vagal nerve stimulation (VNS), which so far has shown improvements in ADAS-Cog in studies with small numbers of participants, with several larger trials underway. It is hypothesized that acetylcholine and noradrenaline signaling interact in attentional processes.

Dopamine

Dopamine (DA) is important for encoding of memories and hippocampal plasticity. Degeneration of dopaminergic neurons and dysregulation of dopaminergic signalling have been found in AD. In the Effects of Dopaminergic Therapy in Patients with Alzheimer's Disease (DOPAD) phase II trial, transdermal rotigotine was compared to placebo at 24 weeks in patients with probable AD[34]. Rotigotine is a dopamine agonist, primarily at D1/D2/D3 receptors. No changes were seen in the ADAS-Cog, however ADLs and FAB measures were improved. Caution should be noted with use of dopaminergic agents with regards to worsening of neuropsychiatric symptoms, in particular psychosis, and development of impulse control disorders.

Serotonin

Serotonin (or 5-hydroxytryptamine, 5-HT) is especially important in the regulation of appetite and emotions and may be important for memory. AD patients do not have structural deficits in serotonergic circuits until late in the condition, though some abnormalities of 5-HT receptor density and function have been reported. It has been postulated that this may be important for mood changes in dementia. Trazodone, a serotonin 2A antagonist and reuptake inhibitor, has been shown in a small, propensity matched, longitudinal study over 4 years to slow decline in cognition by 0.5 points a year as measured by the MMSE[35]. The postulated mechanism in this preliminary study is hypothesized to be trazodone's enhancement of slow wave sleep (SWS) rather than specifically related to its serotoninergic effects. During SWS, episodic memories are consolidated and restriction of SWS has been shown to accelerate amyloid beta accumulation in preclinical models.

Other neurotransmitters

γ-aminobutyric acid (GABA) is the main neurotransmitter mediating inhibition in the nervous system. Compared to the impairments found in glutamatergic and cholinergic systems, fewer consistent alterations in GABAergic neurotransmission have been found in AD.

Histaminergic neurons projecting from the hypothalamic tuberomammillary nucleus mediate a variety of physiological functions, including sleep and homeostatic processes. There is a loss of histaminergic neurons in AD. So far, preclinical pharmaceutical development efforts have focused on antagonism or inverse agonism (reduces baseline levels of receptor signalling) of histamine receptor 3 (H3R), a presynaptic autoreceptor and agonism of histamine receptor 4.

Adenosine receptors are widespread in neural, microglial, and astroglial tissue. Adenosine levels and receptor density has been found to be reduced in AD. Key adenosine receptors are the A1 and A2 receptors, of which caffeine is a non-selective antagonist. Preclinical development efforts have so far focused on adenosine receptor antagonists, including Istradefylline, an adenosine 2A receptor antagonist which is used in Parkinson's disease to reduce 'off' periods (i.e. when levodopa has worn off).

Further reading

The cholinergic hypothesis

Hampel H, Mesulam M-M, Cuello AC, et al. The cholinergic system in the pathophysiology and treatment of Alzheimer's disease. Brain. 2018;141(7):1917–1933.

Neurochemistry of agitation in Alzheimer's disease. Overall, the authors found monoaminergic dysfunction, but with relative noradrenergic postsynaptic hyperactivity.

Liu KY, Stringer AE, Reeves SJ, et al. The neurochemistry of agitation in Alzheimer's disease: A systematic review. Ageing Res Rev. 2018 May;43:99–107.

Neuropathology in non-Alzheimer dementias

Neuropathology of VaD

The German-Austrian psychiatrist Theodore Meynert, after which the cholinergic forebrain nucleus is named, believed that abnormal blood flow was critical to the pathogenesis of dementia. Some of the earliest efforts to find medications to treat dementia focused on vasodilatory action.

In VaD, the original descriptions of pathology revolved around large cerebral infarctions resulting in cognitive and functional impairment, either by sheer volume loss or by strategic positioning. It is increasingly accepted that more progressive accumulation of vascular change can cause damage without evidence of discrete infarction. Large infarctions usually affect the cerebral cortex and underlying white matter, usually in watershed areas (areas at the end of the blood supply territory of different arteries) and are sometimes associated with lacunes (small cavities). Microinfarcts are lesions usually less than 2 mm in diameter. White matter changes have been described extensively in dementia and were considered rare before the development of methods to image the brain but are now considered central to the understanding of cerebral VaD. The term Binswanger's disease and leukoaraiosis have been used to describe white matter abnormalities best seen on MRI and these are universal in people with VaD and very common in people with AD.

Neuropathology in DLB

The pathology of DLB consists of Lewy bodies in the neocortex. The Lewy body was described a century ago; refinements in staining and increased interest have focused attention on this piece of pathology. It is an intracellular neuronal inclusion body consisting in large part of aggregated, filamentous alpha-synuclein and other constituents including ubiquitin and neurofilaments. In Parkinson's disease, Lewy bodies are typically found in the substantia nigra, locus coeruleus, and in the nucleus basalis of Meynert. In DLB they are found much more diffusely, including in the frontal and temporal cortex, hence the term 'cortical Lewy body disease'.

Fronto-temporal dementia

Fronto-temporal dementia (FTD) is a term referring to dementia where there is predominant degeneration of the frontal and temporal lobes. FTD is the fourth most common type of dementia[36]. In general, these dementias have an earlier onset than AD and are usually present from age 60 onwards. Put simply, FTD can be subdivided into behavioural variant FTD (bvFTD), which presents with frontal symptoms, and primary progressive aphasia (PPA), which presents with language deficits. A diverse array of underlying pathologies cause FTD, including mutations in the *MAPT, GRN, FUS, and TARDBP* genes, and in chromosome 9 open reading frame 72 (C9orf72).

In bvFTD, degeneration of right-sided, frontal regions causes a frontal-dysexecutive syndrome including disinhibition, apathy, and compulsivity. The main features are insidious onset and slow progression, early loss of personal and social awareness, early signs of disinhibition, hyperorality, stereotyped behaviour, distractibility, and emotional changes. Spatial orientation and praxis are relatively preserved.

In PPA, degeneration of mainly left-sided, temporal structures leads to deficits in understanding the meaning of words (semantic variant), or in grammar (non-fluent/agrammatic variant) or difficulty with word-finding (logopenic variant, from Greek 'loss of words'). Logopenic variant PPA (lvPPA) is almost always caused by an underlying Alzheimer's disease process. Non-fluent aphasia can also be seen in corticobasal syndrome (CBS) and progressive supranuclear palsy (PSP).

Cognitive testing: The Frontal Assessment Battery (FAB) can be useful in distinguishing AD from FTD or other conditions with frontal dysexecutive syndromes (e.g. Parkinson's plus syndromes). It consists of six questions, including the Luria (fist–edge–palm) test (see Fig. 2.36).

Investigations: structural MRI, see imaging sections for functional imaging in FTD.

Management: As for AD, non-pharmacological measures and support with daily living may be required. There is little evidence for any pharmacological strategies to manage cognitive symptoms. SSRIs, trazodone, atypical antipsychotics, and time-limited courses of benzodiazepines are often used for BPSD in FTD.

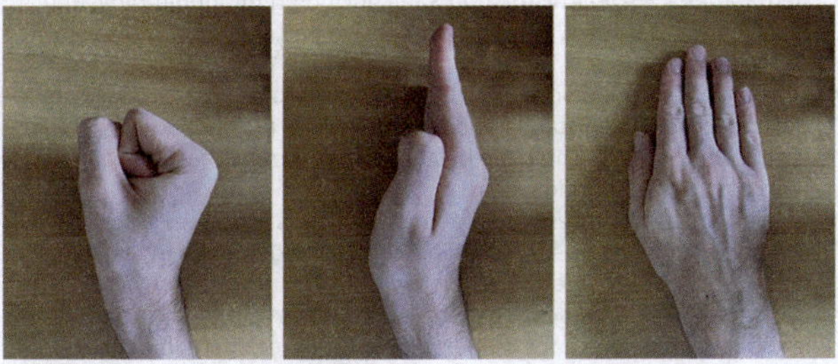

Fig. 2.36 Luria's fist–edge–palm (FEP) test.

The examiner demonstrates the sequence three times. Then the examiner asks the participant to perform the sequence together three times. The participant then is asked to demonstrate it alone. Six consecutive series alone scores 3, three consecutive series alone scores 2, and being able to only perform the series with the examiner scores 1.

Assessment scales

It is becoming increasingly common to carry out formal ratings in clinical practice. In clinic, commonly used scales include the MoCA, ACE-III, or MMSE. Some have been used more commonly in research studies, for example the ADAS, Clinical Dementia Rating (CDR), and CERAD. It is important to understand why the scales are being used. None are diagnostic, many are used to screen for a condition, or to monitor progress in treatment. Some of the more commonly used scales are as follows:

- The Montreal Cognitive Assessment (MoCA): Widely used in memory clinics. Normal controls score between 25.2 and 29.6 out of 30, with a suggested cutoff of < 26 for MCI or AD.
- The Mini Mental State Examination (MMSE): Scored out of 30, and tests the domains of orientation, language, writing, memory, and praxis. Cutoff is 24. Less sensitive than other scales for detecting MCI.
- Addenbrooke's Cognitive Examination (ACE-III): A longer scale which covers cognitive domains in more depth, often used to detect more subtle deficits if not picked up on the MoCA[37].
- Informant Questionnaire on Cognitive Decline in the Elderly (IQCODE) evaluates how patients compare to 10 years ago. In the 16 item version, each item is scored from 1 (much improved) to 5 (much worse) and the average score calculated (e.g. an average of 3 suggests no change).
- Alzheimer's Disease Assessment Scale (ADAS): This is now a standard cognitive scale for drug trials. It assesses a number of cognitive functions including memory, language, and praxis and it also has a section devoted to non-cognitive features.
- Clock-face drawing test: This is a popular test, particularly in primary care as it is easy to administer and is less threatening to patients (Fig. 2.37).
- Clinical Dementia Rating: The CDR is probably the most widely used global scale to give an overall severity rating in dementia, ranging from 0 (none), 0.5 (questionable dementia), through mild and moderate to severe dementia. Each is rated in six domains—memory, orientation, judgement and problem solving, community affairs, home and hobbies, and personal care.
- The Consortium to Establish a Registry for Alzheimer's Disease (CERAD) battery has a 35-year history of usage, including for longitudinal and interventional studies. This comprehensive battery has a total score (TS) of 100.
- Global Deterioration Scale: The Global Deterioration Scale consists of the description of seven stages of dementia from 1 (normal) to 7 where all verbal ability is lost. The scale has been used extensively and validated with post-mortem findings.
- Cornell scale for depression in dementia: This is a 19-item scale which specifically assesses depression in people with dementia in five main domains—mood-related signs, behavioural disturbance, physical signs, cyclic functions, and ideation disturbance. A mixture of informant-rated and observational ratings makes it ideal for assessment in patients with cognitive impairment where information from the patient might not always be available. A score of 8 or above suggests significant depressive symptoms.

Examples of clock face drawing

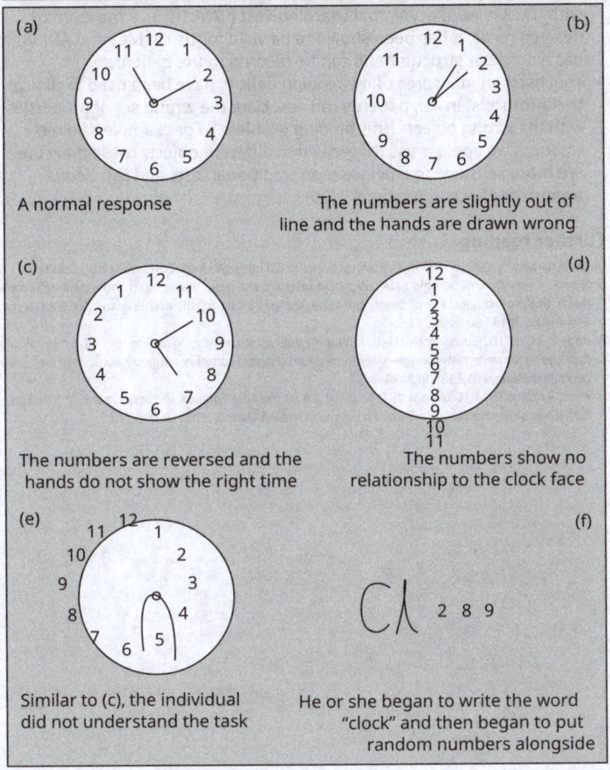

Fig. 2.37 Examples of clock-face drawing.
Reproduced from Burns, Downs, Kampers, *Current dementia*, Current Medicine Group, 2003. With kind permission.

- Neuropsychiatric Inventory (NPI): Twelve behavioural areas are assessed in the NPI (delusions, hallucinations, agitation, depression, anxiety, euphoria, apathy, disinhibition, irritability, aberrant motor behaviour, night-time behaviours, and appetite/eating disorders), each of which is rated on a four-point scale of frequency and a three-point scale of severity. Distress in carers is also measured.
- Bristol Activities of Daily Living Scale (BADLS): A 20-item scale rated on severity looking at basic ADLs (e.g. feeding, eating, and toileting) and instrumental ADLs (which refer to the performance of more complex tasks such as shopping, travelling, answering the telephone, and handling finances).

- The NIH Toolbox Cognition Battery (NIHTB-CB) is designed to be a quick and easily administered touchscreen digital battery. When combined with the Rey Auditory Verbal Learning Test (RAVLT-DR), a measure of delayed recall, it has been shown to be valid for use in MCI and AD[38] It has a modular structure and can be tailored to the patient.
- Touchscreen measures of misbinding deficits have been used in clinical trial protocols. In AD, patients can associate the wrong set of properties with the wrong objects (the 'binding problem'). For example, the red colour of an apple is associated with a different object. These measures are more sensitive to changes than traditional tests and can detect treatment effects more quickly[39].

Further reading

Burns A, Lawlor B, Craig S (1999). *Assessment scales in old age psychiatry*. London, Martin Dunitz.

Breton A, Casey D, Arnaoutoglou NA. Cognitive tests for the detection of mild cognitive impairment (MCI), the prodromal stage of dementia: Meta-analysis of diagnostic accuracy studies. Int J Geriatr Psychiatry. 2019 Feb;34(2):233–242.

Pertzov Y, Miller TD, Gorgoraptis N, et al. Binding deficits in memory following medial temporal lobe damage in patients with voltage-gated potassium channel complex antibody-associated limbic encephalitis. Brain. 2013;136(8):2474–2485.

Hackett K, Krikorian R, Giovannetti T, et al. Utility of the NIH Toolbox for assessment of prodromal Alzheimer's disease and dementia. Alzheimers Dement (Amst). 2018;10:764–772.

Risk factors for dementia

For most presentations of dementia, there are no commonly testable genetic anormalities which are proven risk factors for dementia. Early-onset genetic types are associated with abnormalities in the amyloid precursor protein (chromosome 21) and also presenilin 1 (chromosome 14) and presenilin 2 (chromosome 1). Late-onset sporadic Alzheimer's disease is associated with the presence of *APOE e4* (chromosome 19). See the section *Genetics of AD* in this chapter for more information about genetic risk factors and genetic testing. Other relatively well-supported risk factors include raised cholesterol, raised blood pressure, diabetes, history of myocardial infarction as well as the risk factors traditionally associated with dementia in epidemiological studies such as head injury, depression, and thyroid disease. Recent epidemiological evidence suggests that the following are important exposures to consider: physical inactivity, current smoking, depression, low education, diabetes, midlife obesity, midlife hypertension, and hearing loss[40]. It is clear that new modalities (e.g. amyloid PET) to detect Alzheimer pathology well before clinical declaration of the disease may alter our understanding of risk for dementia.

Further reading

Nianogo RA, Rosenwohl-Mack A, Yaffe K, et al. Risk factors associated with Alzheimer disease and related dementias by sex and race and ethnicity in the US. JAMA Neurol. 2022 Jun 1;79(6):584–591.

Management of dementia: an overview

The management of dementia can be viewed in several ways and Figure 2.38 summarizes the main treatments available in relation to the major symptoms.

At diagnosis, in addition to information giving, patients are usually directed to local support services and asked to consider practical issues with their families such as driving, legal, and financial matters. The use of easy-to-use calendars and simple memory support strategies are often helpful. Examples of other non-pharmacological measures include cognitive stimulation therapy, group reminiscence approaches, and cognitive rehabilitation, in addition to maintaining a healthy lifestyle.

Symptomatic treatments are generally directed towards psychiatric symptoms and behavioural problems.

The following antidementia drugs are the most widely prescribed globally:

- Cholinergic agents:
  - Donepezil (Aricept®) 5–10 mg daily dose
  - Rivastigmine (Exelon®) 6–12 mg daily dose
  - Galantamine (Reminyl®) 8–24 mg daily dose
- Glutamatergic agent:
  - Memantine (Ebixa®) 10–20 mg daily dose

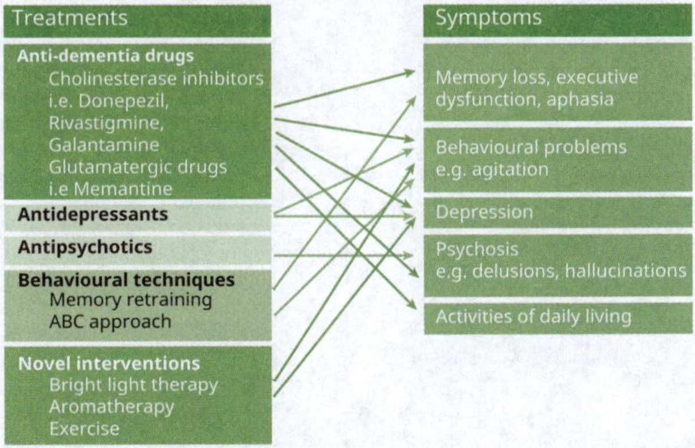

Fig. 2.38 Management of dementia.

The antidementia drugs are used to moderate the course of the illness and different strategies have been described, as outlined in Figure 2.39, to stabilize the decline (by slowing progression or even arresting it) or to provide symptomatic improvement which eventually wears off.

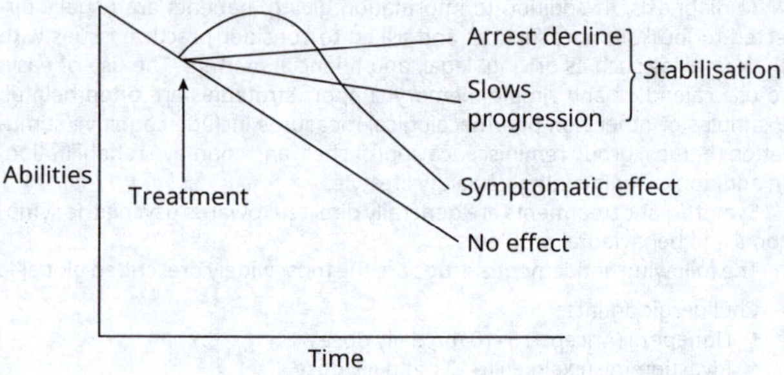

Fig. 2.39 Progress in treatment.

The cholinergic system and cholinesterase inhibitors

These drugs work on the cholinergic system by inhibiting the enzyme (acetylcholinesterase, AChE) which breaks down acetylcholine into choline and acetate (see Fig. 2.40). There are also cholinergic drugs which act directly on the muscarinic and nicotinic receptors, but these have generally been found to be disappointing therapeutically.

Early biochemical studies demonstrated a diminution of cholinergic neurotransmission in the brains of people with AD and led to studies aimed at replacement. Lecithin was trialled in the expectation that it would increase the levels of choline (it is converted in the body to choline, which itself is unpalatable when ingested directly and gives rise to severe gastrointestinal side effects). Placebo-controlled trials showed some improvements in cognition, but these were not particularly striking. Tacrine (tetrahydroaminoacridine (THA), an anaesthetic agent and powerful cholinesterase inhibitor used sometimes to reverse post-anaesthetic delirium) was shown to be superior to placebo in AD in the mid-1980s. The drug required dosing 4 times a day and was toxic to the liver, with the majority of people experiencing significant gastrointestinal side effects. The better-tolerated donepezil, rivastigmine, and galantamine are more acceptable alternatives to tacrine.

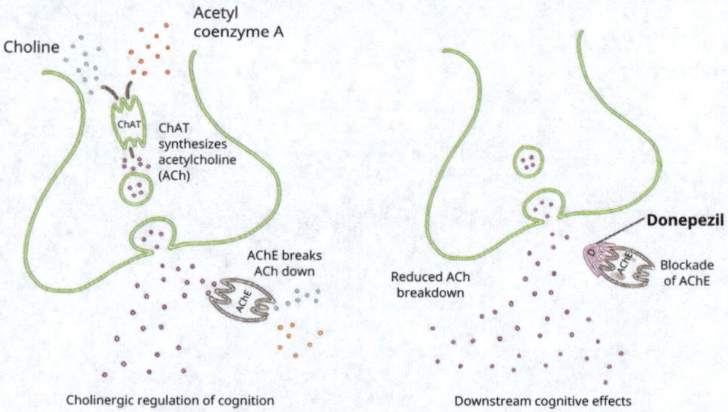

Fig. 2.40 Acetylcholine synthesis in the brain. The enzyme choline acetyl-transferase (ChAT) produces acetylcholine. The enzyme acetylcholinesterase (AChE) breaks it down. Cholinesterase inhibitors, like donepezil, block AChE leading to reduced breakdown of acetylcholine and downstream cognitive effects.

Specific treatments available for AD—the acetylcholinesterase inhibitors (AChEIs)

- **Donepezil** (Aricept®): its characteristics include: high oral bioavailability which is unaffected by food; a long plasma half-life of 70 hours permitting once-daily dosing; almost total plasma protein binding; highly selective reversible inhibition of acetylcholinesterase. Pivotal studies all show an improvement in both cognition and clinician-rated improvement with a greater effect of the 10 mg dose compared with 5 mg. The most common side effects of donepezil are understandable in terms of the peripheral (as opposed to central nervous system) mechanism of action and are largely gastrointestinal, including nausea, vomiting, diarrhoea, and anorexia. Some patients develop muscle cramps, headache, dizziness, syncope, or flushing. Haematological side effects include anaemia and thrombocytopenia, and cardiac side effects may be seen including bradyarrhythmia and syncope. Other side effects include headache, insomnia, weakness, drowsiness, fatigue, and agitation.
- **Rivastigmine** (Exelon®) has an effect both on acetylcholinesterase and butyrylcholinesterase. It has a short half-life compared with donepezil (2 h). Because of its short half-life it needs to be given twice a day, and it requires slow titration to minimize the cholinergic side effects. The trial data suggest a similar side-effect profile to donepezil, including nausea, vomiting, and anorexia. It has become available as a transdermal patch allowing for a novel once-daily administration, but is also useful in allowing treatment in some patients who cannot accept oral route. Rivastigmine also has an indication for the treatment of Parkinson's-associated dementia.
- **Galantamine** has a dual action as an AChEI and with a modulating effect on nicotinic receptors. It has the expected tolerability problems in keeping with other AChEIs, the majority being gastrointestinal. It has a half-life between that of donepezil and rivastigmine. It can be given once or twice daily and has an optimal dose of between 16 mg and 24 mg/day. It can be given with food due to its greater than 90% bioavailability. The effect size for the three drugs is essentially similar. The main contraindications are asthma and cardiac conduction disorders.

Antidementia drug prescribing—the practicalities

The AChEIs are statistically and clinically superior to placebo in improving cognitive deficits, global ratings of dementia, and ADLs in AD. What is also evident is that higher doses are consistently more effective than lower doses. A meta analysis of 80 trials suggests that the treatment effect is approximately 1 point on the MMSE at 3, 6, and 12 months after starting treatment[41]. Interestingly, the effect was found to be double in LBD. To put this in context, a decline of 4–5 points on the MMSE would be expected over 12 months without any treatment.

When a patient who has only recently started treatment doesn't appear to be responding to an AChEI, switching to another cholinesterase inhibitor is unlikely to be beneficial (but possible due to individual variability) and the best strategy is to optimize the dose and then consider adding memantine if there is still no response.

Longitudinal data suggest that the positive effects of cholinesterase inhibitors can last many years[42]. The risks and benefits of stopping must be discussed fully with the patient and carer. Clinicians often find that stopping an AChEI in a patient leads to an unexpected deterioration of behaviour (e.g. increased agitation) or cognition, proving the drug was having more of an effect that realized. When attempting withdrawal it is important to monitor closely for any deterioration so the medication can be reinstated quickly and the same level of symptomatic effect can be regained.

Memantine for AD

Memantine, a partial glutamate receptor antagonist, is used in the treatment of moderate to severe AD. Glutamate, an excitatory amino acid neurotransmitter, is found diffusely in the cortex and hippocampus and is excessively available in a number of conditions including AD. Memantine acts to block the effect of glutamate at NMDA receptors. It has been available in Germany for over 30 years for various neurological symptoms and cognitive impairment. Early evidence for a role for memantine in dementia was in VaD and in moderate to severe AD. The treatment effect size of memantine is less than for cholinesterase inhibitors[42].

The initial dose is 5 mg once a day which should be increased in 5 mg increments at intervals of at least 1 week until a maximum dose of 10 mg twice a day is reached, or 20 mg in a single daily dose. Memantine is generally better tolerated than the cholinesterase inhibitors. The most common adverse events of memantine include dizziness, headaches, fatigue, diarrhoea, and gastric pain. In clinical experience the side effects which are most likely to lead to discontinuation are restlessness and hyperexcitation. There are very few cholinergic side effects. Currently memantine is predominantly used in the treatment of moderate to severe AD when it is felt that cholinesterase inhibitors are no longer effective. In these circumstances, memantine can be prescribed alongside the existing cholinesterase inhibitor (combination therapy). Memantine has a role as an alternative to AChEIs in the treatment of patients with mild to moderate AD who are either unable to tolerate AChEIs or when AChEIs are contraindicated, e.g. problems with cardiac conduction or severe asthma.

Emerging therapeutics for AD

Emerging therapies in AD

A multitude of new therapeutics are in development for Alzheimer's disease and a recent review suggests the following categories: disease-modifying biologics, disease-modifying small molecules, symptomatic cognitive enhancers, and therapies for neuropsychiatric symptoms. Additionally, there has been significant innovation in medical device-based neuromodulation treatments. Below we highlight some examples, see section on *BPSD for neuropsychiatric treatments* and further reading below for in depth coverage of the field.

Anti-amyloid biologics

The anti-amyloid therapies are monoclonal antibodies which target amyloid in the brain. The concept is to treat intensively initially to reduce the level of amyloid below a key threshold (the measurement unit being centiloids), after which it can be kept low with less frequent dosing. Overall, these biologics are very good at reducing amyloid, however, this does not necessarily translate into a commensurate level of clinical improvement. Overall, a delay in progression of 3–5.3 months has been observed over an 18-month dosing schedule[43]. See below for efficacy of selected drugs. Confounders include copathology, such as limbic-predominant age-related TDP-43 encephalopathy (LATE) and the fact that patients may need to be observed for longer than standard treatment trials to observe larger changes in outcomes.

As large molecule biologics, these drugs must be administered by intravenous infusion. Biologic infusion clinics exist in other specialties, for example gastroenterology and oncology, and require regular patient visits and specialist nursing staff. Difficult peripheral intravenous cannulation (DPIVC) is estimated at 10–24% of adults[44]. In future, from a pharmaceutical development perspective, subcutaneous formulations may offer greater convenience and patient choice.

Side effects include amyloid-related imaging abnormalities (ARIAs), which is a term that encompasses oedema and haemorrhage. These occur as a by-product of removing amyloid from the brain. Whilst most are not significant, a small percentage are more serious.

Neuromodulation

Brain stimulation is an emerging strategy in treating neurocognitive disorders. Neuromodulation approaches can be divided into non-invasive brain stimulation (NIBS), which can be administered in an outpatient setting, and invasive approaches which require neurosurgery, such as deep brain stimulation (DBS). In general, these approaches are thought to work on a systems level by modulating functional connectivity of key cognitive networks, and biologically by inducing neuroplasticity.

There are several reasons why interest has grown in neuromodulation, the first being technical advances in commercially available systems. A key benefit of these approaches is the ability to target and tailor treatment using patient-specific neuroimaging. For NIBS, the targeted nature of treatment means that there are generally fewer side effects than for pharmacotherapies which can have widespread physiological effects, or in the case of anti-amyloid treatments, ARIAs. Additionally, neuromodulation treatments tend to be time limited, or applied episodically to response whereas medications tend to be given continuously. Different neuromodulation modalities exist, which originate from fundamental research methods used in cognitive neuroscience.

However, invasive brain stimulation in contrast does carry the risks of the required neurosurgical intervention. For both NIBS and invasive brain stimulation, another consideration is the cost of equipment and expertise required for administration.

So far, emerging neuromodulation approaches have been used in conjunction with standard cholinergic therapy, however, analogous to transcranial magnetic stimulation (TMS) in the depressive disorders, it may also find a niche for those who cannot tolerate medications. Invasive brain stimulation is likely to remain a last line option. So far, key targets for DBS include the fornix, nucleus basalis of Meynert (NBM), the ventral capsule and striatum.

Further reading

A review of new pharmacotherapies

Cummings J, Lee G, Nahed P, et al. Alzheimer's disease drug development pipeline: 2022. Alzheimers Dement (NY). 2022;8(1):e12295.

The TRAILBLAZER-ALZ 2 trial (donanemab)[45]

Sims JR, Zimmer JA, Evans CD, et al. Donanemab in early symptomatic Alzheimer disease: The TRAILBLAZER-ALZ 2 Randomized Clinical Trial. JAMA. 2023;330(6):512–527.

CLARITY AD trial (lecanemab) [46]

van Dyck CH, Swanson CJ, Aisen P, et al. Lecanemab in early Alzheimer's disease. N Engl J Med. 2022;388(1):9–21.

ENGAGE and EMERGE (aducanumab)[47]

Budd Haeberlein S, Aisen PS, Barkhof F, et al. Two randomized phase 3 studies of aducanumab in early Alzheimer's disease. J Prev Alzheimers Dis. 2022;9(2):197–210.

Non-invasive brain stimulation (Transcranial Pulse Stimulation)[48]

Beisteiner R, Matt E, Fan C, et al. Transcranial pulse stimulation with ultrasound in Alzheimer's disease: A new navigated focal brain therapy. Adv Sci (Weinh). 2020 Feb;7(3):1902583.

A review of Deep Brain Stimulation (DBS)[49]

Luo Y, Sun Y, Tian X, et al. Deep brain stimulation for Alzheimer's disease: Stimulation parameters and potential mechanisms of action [Review]. Front Aging Neurosci. 2021 March;11:13.

Drug treatment in non-Alzheimer dementias

Vascular cognitive impairment

The main focus here is primary and secondary prevention by controlling risk events to reduce vascular events. Early identification and treatment of hypertension, which is also a risk factor for AD, has been shown to reduce the risk of dementia among patients who have experienced stroke. Lipid-lowering medications are also important in secondary prevention of stroke and may also protect against dementia. Other factors which are crucial in reducing the risk of VaD are aerobic exercise, stopping smoking, weight reduction, control of atrial fibrillation with anticoagulation, and nutritional education.

There is a treatment effect of AChEIs in patients with mixed dementias. AChEIs, however, are still not licensed for the treatment of pure VCI. Generally, in pure VCI, they are not routinely prescribed because the magnitude of the effect may only be small[50]. Cholinergic structures are vulnerable to ischaemic changes which can lead to significant loss of cholinergic neurotransmission, although rarely to the magnitude seen in AD. A recent Cochrane network meta-analysis found that there was the most evidence for donepezil 10 mg, and for galantamine, with less evidence for rivastigmine. The authors concluded that 'the effect is modest, but in the absence of any other treatments, people living with VCI may still wish to consider the use of these agents'.

Dementia with Lewy bodies

Cognition

Cholinesterase inhibitors have been shown to benefit patients with LBD, with a treatment effect approximately double of that seen in AD. AChEIs have not been found to worsen the motor symptoms of Parkinson's disease. Rivastigmine has a licence for PD dementia in the USA and UK, and donepezil has a licence for DLB in Japan. Donepezil has been associated with fewer adverse effects than rivastigmine. There is less evidence for galantamine overall. Memantine is another option which can be considered. Its effect size is modest and it is mainly an alternative to ACHEIs when these cannot be used.

BPSD in LBD

The dosage of any dopaminergic medicines which the patient are taking should be reviewed. Cholinesterase inhibitors (most evidence for donepezil) and memantine are recommended above antipsychotics for treatment of neuropsychiatric symptoms, including psychotic symptoms. Use of antipsychotics is complicated by the fact that they block dopamine receptors and therefore can worsen parkinsonism. If needed, quetiapine and clozapine are most often used in LBD because they are least likely to worsen parkinsonism. The FDA-approved atypical antipsychotic pimavanserin is specifically indicated for Parkinson's disease psychosis. Pimavanersin is an inverse agonist (i.e. reduces levels of signaling to below baseline) at the 5-HT2A receptor and interestingly, is an antipsychotic with no D2 antagonist action. This means that it does not worsen parkinsonism.

Further reading

Taylor JP, McKeith IG, Burn DJ, et al. New evidence on the management of Lewy body dementia. Lancet Neurol. 2020 Feb;19(2):157–169 **[51]**

Guidelines and managing dementia

Millions of people across the world and up to 1 million in the UK have dementia. The history of therapeutics in dementia has been one of prolonged effort followed by limited but significant breakthroughs. These have inevitably led to huge demand for treatments but also a much more systematic approach to making diagnoses available across a wider proportion of the at-risk population. The newly developed disease-modifying treatments like aducanumab, lecanamab, and donanemab will challenge healthcare systems to a much greater extent than the advent of AChEIs did. AChEIs drove provision of memory clinics with routine availability of now widely available imaging (CT or MRI). The need to establish presence of amyloid and ability of PET to pick up these deposits well before a clinical syndrome of dementia has established itself, will mean that a wholesale re-engineering of old age psychiatry and memory services will be needed. Along with this will be high demand for PET scans—given that the UK has under 100 of these scanners in 2023, rationing access will be needed.

Across many countries, guidelines have been developed for healthcare organizations on managing dementia. In the UK, National Institute for Health and Care Excellence (NICE) guidance has been very important in driving availability of medications. At some points the UK has gone further and made results of NICE technology appraisals legally binding rather than just a recommendation. Decisions in many countries about future dementia treatments will be inevitably political—they will involve considerations of cost versus benefit.

The most recent NICE guidance on managing dementia is 2018.[1] Key principles are:

- Involving people with dementia in decisions about their care.
- Primary care assessment should lead to referral to memory clinics or, if history is of rapid progression, to neurology clinic.
- Diagnosis of AD should follow established criteria, involve a test of episodic verbal memory, and if structural imaging leaves issue unclear, advanced investigations like FDG-PET, perfusion SPECT, or CSF testing.
- Newly diagnosed patients receive post-diagnosis counselling and follow-up.
- Cognitive stimulation therapy should be offered (relatively rarely used in practice).
- Use cholinesterase inhibitors for mild to moderate cases of AD, and memantine for severe AD, or if AChEIs not tolerated in mild to moderate cases. AChEIs should not be stopped because AD advances.
- Manage non-cognitive symptoms in structured fashion—no more than 6 weeks on antipsychotics, do not use valproate, melatonin, or antidepressants routinely.
- Ensure good care for non-dementia symptoms like pain and falls.
- Use palliative approach in advanced dementia; do not use enteral feeding unless reversible.
- Support carers and train and educate staff caring for people with dementia.
- Minimize moves for people with dementia.

Reference

NICE (2018). Dementia: assessment, management and support for people living with dementia and their carers NG97

Management of behavioural and psychological symptoms of dementia: 1, Approaches

- Behavioural and psychological symptoms of dementia (BPSD) symptom clusters span the usual psychiatric diagnostic hierarchy including psychosis (delusions and hallucinations), depression, anxiety, sleeping and eating disturbances. There may be anxious obsessions and compulsions. Features more specific to BPSD include agitation, aggression, irritability, disinhibition, and apathy. Patients' capacity for empathy may be lessened and their personality changed.
- All patients with dementia will naturally experience some of these BPSD during the course of their dementia and many may be time limited.
- Several scales exist to measure BPSD and treatment response. General measures include the Clinical Global Impression scores of Change and Severity (CGI-C, CGI-S), the Neuropsychiatric Inventory (NPI), the Behavioural Pathology in Alzheimer's Disease (BEHAVE-AD), and the Neurobehavioral Rating Scale (NBRS). Domain-specific scales which have also appeared in recent key trials of pharmacotherapies include the Cohen–Mansfield Agitation Inventory (CMAI), the Scale for the Assessment of Positive Symptoms–Hallucinations and Delusions (SAPS–H+D), and the Cornell Scale for Depression in Dementia.
- Non-pharmacological treatments can be effective first-line treatments for many people with behavioural problems associated with dementia[52].
- Multisensory stimulation using different sensory modalities has been found to be helpful, as has music therapy. Another type of therapeutic intervention is massage therapy, which can be relaxing. Aromatherapy has been used for a number of years for a variety of health problems, the most common agents being lemon balm or lavender. These can be either given through skin application or by inhalation. Active agents in aromatherapy oils have been identified (the terpines) which cross the blood–brain barrier easily because of their lipid solubility. Bright light therapy has also been trialled for BPSD. There is some evidence to suggest that bright light might have a calming influence over and above any antidepressant effect (the latter being a well-documented effect of bright light, which at an extreme can lead to a 'manic switch'). Time spent with animals ('pet therapy') has also been used to create a positive emotional environment. Looking back at old photos, or reflecting on happy memories ('reminiscence therapy') is another positive intervention.
- Depression occurs commonly in people with dementia, some reports even suggesting it is a universal phenomenon. A significant clinical depression can occur in up to half or two-thirds of patients and is said to be commoner in VaD and DLB. Psychosocial interventions should be a first step where possible.

- Apathy is being increasingly recognized as a key symptom experienced by patients. The *ADMET 2* trial showed a beneficial effect of methylphenidate in AD when measured on the NPI apathy subscale, and clinical global impression scores. Additionally, other noradrenergic agents, such as atomoxetine or SNRIs could be considered. Box 2.5 summarizes the management of BPSD.

Box 2.5 Management of BPSD (behavioural and psychological symptoms of dementia)

- Define what the problem or symptom to be addressed is.
- Determine if there is a simple medical problem explaining the symptom. For example, is it a transient feature of delirium explained by an infection or recent hip surgery? Is there pain not being verbally reported (e.g. resistive and angry patient when examined, increased pulse or blood pressure when touched).
- Decide if an independent psychiatric disorder like severe depressive disorder or psychotic illness may explain the symptom and warrant independent treatment, such as antidepressants and/or antipsychotics.
- Is there a clear sensory or environmental factor worsening the problem, e.g. deafness, darkness, recent change of ward.
- If these issues have been addressed, do we still need to intervene to manage the problem/symptom?

Further reading

Scales K, Zimmerman S, Miller SJ. Evidence-based nonpharmacological practices to address behavioral and psychological symptoms of dementia. Gerontologist. 2018 Jan 18;58(suppl_1):S88–102.

Management of BPSD: 2, Medication choice

- Whilst non-pharmacological therapeutic interventions remain the cornerstone approach to the behavioural and psychological symptoms in AD, there are cases where psychotropic medication is required. Medication should be reserved for cases where all other interventions have failed, but clinical experience suggests frequent and early requests to clinicians for prescriptions. The target symptom-based approach is the gold standard and this involves matching the most salient target symptoms to a relevant drug class.
- It is therefore imperative to always define the true cause of the behaviour and when drug intervention is required, adopt the 'start low and go slow' approach with the chosen antipsychotic and use the simplest dosage regimen possible.

Cognitive enhancers

- Optimizing antidementia treatment can be helpful in managing BPSD. Cholinesterase inhibitors can be helpful for dysphoria and anxiety symptoms, but they have been shown not to be effective for routine aggression and agitation in dementia. Memantine has a moderate effect on agitation and delusions. Memantine can be added for this indication onto existing cholinesterase therapy.

Antipsychotics

The antipsychotics as a group can show benefit for agitation associated with psychotic features and may also show benefit for agitation or aggression not associated with psychotic features. The primary efficacy is similar for all neuroleptics but the side effects and induced tolerance of these drugs are variable. They are certainly effective in treating agitation and restlessness; there have been a number of meta-analyses of the literature showing that in patients with AD, neuroleptics are effective in controlling agitation, and that about 20% of patients will gain extra benefit from these. More recent studies have concentrated on AD, whereas many earlier studies also included patients with acute confusional states (delirium). There are no absolute rules on dosage—generally one should use a lower dose than one might in a psychotic patient who did not have cognitive impairment. The side effects are well known and are probably more exaggerated in patients who have dementia—extrapyramidal signs, tardive dyskinesia (in up to 50% of patients), postural hypotension, sedation (due to blockage of histamine receptors), anticholinergic effects, agranulocytosis, liver and cardiac toxicity. Neuroleptics are likely to cause higher mortality and morbidity in patients with DLB. With regard to the specific agents that can be used, there may be little to choose between the main neuroleptics and, as with other drugs, choice is determined often on the basis of familiarity. The main concern has been about the apparent increased risk of cerebrovascular events and of death among patients with dementia prescribed these agents in trials. The risks appear robustly supported and clinicians prescribing antipsychotics in the presence of dementia need to show clear reasons why they believe the risks are outweighed by the benefits.

Example medication choices: clinician choices should be tailored to the patient's symptoms and particular medical history and circumstances. Cautious doses of risperidone (0.25–0.5 mg BD), olanzapine or aripiprazole are reasonable. Risperidone is approved for short-term (6 weeks) treatment of persistent aggression on the context of AD. There is less evidence for quetiapine but it may be useful in DLB. Brexpiprazole has been approved specifically by the FDA for agitation associated with AD.

- A number of non-neuroleptic drugs are also used in the management of patients with dementia. Benzodiazepines are often used for acute sedation but there is limited long-term evidence and an increased mortality risk if used as the core therapy for BPSD. There is limited evidence for mood stabilizers.
- Meta-analytical studies have not found antidepressants to be that effective for depression *per se* in dementia, however there is significant heterogeneity of studies[53]. Generally, SSRIs have been used as a first-line treatment. Citalopram improved agitation in the CitAD trial as measured by the NBRS agitation subscale[54]. Sometimes mirtazapine or trazodone is used for their sedative qualities. Other options include SNRIs and vortioxetine. Agomelatine utilizes a different mechanism of action to most other antidepressants and can be useful in the case of adverse events (AEs) to other classes, but it does require liver function test (LFT) monitoring. In cases of treatment resistance, other antidepressant classes may be used, but note TCAs can have anticholinergic effects.
- *Example medications:* Lorazepam 0.5 mg *pro re nata* (PRN), trazodone 50 mg once per night (ON), and promethazine are commonly encountered in clinical practice acutely for sedation. Citalopram and sertraline are examples of first-line SSRIs, dose adjusted for age. SNRIs include venlafaxine or duloxetine. Bupropion may be helpful for apathy due to its dopaminergic effects. Agomelatine utilizes a melatoninergic mechamism. Its unique mechanism of action avoids some of the side effects of other commonly used ADs but it does require LFT monitoring.
- Pimavanserin is a novel 5-HT2A inverse agonist which is indicated for PD psychotic symptoms, and has also been used in other dementias.
- Other medication choices include prazosin, an alpha-1 blocker, and dextromethorphan-qunidine, which is also used for pseudobulbar affect.
- *Non-invasive brain stimulation:* a systematic review suggests that rTMS may be beneficial for BPSD, especially apathy but longer follow up periods are required[55]. Side effects were found to be mild and transient.

Further reading

Shah A, Lopes AT (2007). Pharmacological interventions for BPSD. In: *Therapeutic strategies in dementia* (ed. CW Ritchie, D Ames, CL Masters, J Cummings), pp. 203226. Oxford, Clinical Publishing.

Are antipsychotics dangerous in dementia?

From the 1980s on, antipsychotics were the mainstay of prescriptions for BPSD. Unlike benzodiazepines, antipsychotics had mounting controlled trial evidence of efficacy for BPSD, including well-designed studies supporting the use of haloperidol, risperidone, and olanzapine. Among those treated with atypical antipsychotics, there appeared to be an advantage of fewer extrapyramidal side effects. Since the 1990s, there have been concerns about the use of these drugs in dementia. Initial concerns focused on over-prescription of these agents, especially among care home residents. In 1997 a prospective study with post-mortem validation[1] suggested that AD patients who had had neuroleptic drugs showed greater pathological and cognitive deterioration. Prescribing fashions change; concern at the time focused on the now-unavailable agent thioridazine.

Since then two arms of evidence have raised concerns. In 2004, the UK Committee for the Safety of Medicines advised all doctors to cease prescribing the atypical antipsychotics risperidone and olanzapine for patients with dementia, due to evidence from controlled trials of increased risk of CVA. There was insufficient evidence to make a confident recommendation about quetiapine. In the USA similar concerns were raised about mortality among patients with dementia prescribed atypical antipsychotics. The debate has broadened; some reports have suggested that risk is equal among older and newer antipsychotics. The evidence of overall increased risk is now widely accepted.

There is, however, little doubt that antipsychotics are among the best supported treatments for BPSD. Confirmation of a possible directly deleterious effect on the progression of the condition has come in later studies of the effect of quetiapine on BPSD in severe institutionalized patients with dementia[2]. Mechanisms of risk are unclear; what is clear is that the risks need to be justified in prescribing these agents for BPSD.

Considerations in prescribing antipsychotic medication for BPSD

- Have non-pharmacological responses to BPSD been considered?
- Have drug treatments other than antipsychotics been tried?
- Is the problem persistent rather than transient?
- What is the cardiovascular risk status of the patient?
- Can cardiovascular risk status be reduced?
- Has the acknowledged risk of cerebrovascular events/fatality been documented and discussed with patient/carers?
- Has a time-limited review of benefits/risks been planned?

References

1. McShane R, Keen J, Gedling K et al. Do neuroleptic drugs hasten cognitive decline in dementia? Prospective study with necropsy follow up. BMJ 1997;314:266–270.
2. Ballard C, Margallo-Lana M, Juszczak E et al. Quetiapine and rivastigmine and cognitive decline in Alzheimer's disease: Randomised double blind placebo controlled trial. BMJ 2005;330:874.

Carers of people with dementia

It is axiomatic to say that caring for a person with dementia is stressful—carers have known that for a long time but it is only relatively recently that the research community has taken this to the next stage.

Problems for carers of people with dementia

- Poverty
- Social isolation
- Anxiety
- Insomnia
- Physical illness

Stress, depression, and anxiety (one-third of carers of those suffering from dementia)

Factors which predict stress in carers include:

- The personality of the carer.
- Poor previous relationship with person with dementia.
- Wandering, insomnia, aggression, and incontinence.
- Dementia rather than non-dementia diagnosis in patient.
- Social isolation.
- Gender (women appear more at risk).

Interventions for carers of people with dementia are ubiquitous, and intervening for the carer cannot, and should not, be distinguished from intervening for the person with dementia. Increased recognition of the morbidity associated with caring for people with dementia has led to increased interest in interventions specifically designed to alleviate carer distress. These are listed below. Evidence for the effectiveness of these interventions is often lacking. Several approaches have been tried, including structured coping programs, exercise, and the use of case managers to help carers coordinate the sometimes complex care arrangements required. Those interventions best supported by evidence include specific care support, cognitive behavioural support, and group-based carer support. A key issue which has been highlighted as more important to carers than medical professionals is managing incontinence, something difficult for the carer to manage and something for which they can be reluctant to ask help. However, incontinence has been associated with a greater likelihood of being admitted to a care home.

Recent guidance suggests that carers of people with dementia should expect:

- An assessment of their needs for respite care and support.
- Tailored psycho-education and skills training.
- Advice on how to look after their own health and well-being.
- Planning advice for the future, including financial issues.

Interventions for carers of people with dementia

- Group carer support
- Practical assistance—care packages
- Day centre care
- Cognitive behavioural therapy
- Interpersonal therapy
- Information/educational courses
- Antidepressant medication

References

1. Barkhof F. Dementia—Role of MRI 2022. Available from: https://radiologyassistant.nl/neuroradiology/dementia/role-of-mri
2. Kolanko MA, Win Z, Loreto F, et al. Amyloid PET imaging in clinical practice. Pract Neurol. 2020 Dec;20(6):451–462.
3. Kanani M-K, Gurunathan N. Misdiagnosis of dementia with Lewy bodies due to venlafaxine. Progress in Neurology and Psychiatry. 2022;26(2):8–10.
4. Bai W, Chen P, Cai H, et al. Worldwide prevalence of mild cognitive impairment among community dwellers aged 50 years and older: a meta-analysis and systematic review of epidemiology studies. Age Ageing. 2022;51(8).
5. Pagnotti RMB, Pudumjee SB, Cross CL, et al. Cognitive and clinical characteristics of patients with limbic-predominant age-related TDP-43 encephalopathy. Neurology. 2023;100(19):e2027–e2035.
6. Laganà V, Bruno F, Altomari N, et al. Neuropsychiatric or behavioral and psychological symptoms of dementia (BPSD): Focus on prevalence and natural history in Alzheimer's disease and frontotemporal dementia. Front Neurol. 2022;13:832199.
7. Iida MA, Farrell K, Walker JM, et al. Predictors of cognitive impairment in primary age-related tauopathy: An autopsy study. Acta Neuropathol Commun. 2021 2021/08/05;9(1):134.
8. Jessen F, Amariglio RE, Buckley RF, et al. The characterisation of subjective cognitive decline. Lancet Neurol. 2020 Mar;19(3):271–278.
9. Jack CR, Jr., Bennett DA, Blennow K, et al. NIA-AA research framework: Toward a biological definition of Alzheimer's disease. Alzheimers Dement. 2018 Apr;14(4):535–562.
10. Dubois B, Villain N, Frisoni GB, et al. Clinical diagnosis of Alzheimer's disease: recommendations of the International Working Group. Lancet Neurol. 2021 Jun;20(6):484–496.
11. Budson A, Solomon, P. (2023). *Memory loss, Alzheimer's disease and dementia.* Heidelberg, Elsevier.
12. Iadecola C, Duering M, Hachinski V, et al. Vascular cognitive impairment and dementia: JACC Scientific Expert Panel. J Am Coll Cardiol. 2019 Jul 2;73(25):3326–3344.
13. Skrobot OA, Black SE, Chen C, et al. Progress toward standardized diagnosis of vascular cognitive impairment: Guidelines from the Vascular Impairment of Cognition Classification Consensus Study. Alzheimers Dement. 2018 Mar;14(3):280–292.
14. Reimers K, Emmert N, Shah H, et al. Capgras-like visual decomposition in Lewy body dementia with therapeutic response to donepezil. Neurol Clin Pract. 2014 Dec;4(6):467–469.
15. Kantarci K, Avula R, Senjem ML, et al. Dementia with Lewy bodies and Alzheimer disease: Neurodegenerative patterns characterized by DTI. Neurology. 2010 Jun 1;74(22):1814–21.
16. Alty J, Cosgrove J, Thorpe D, et al. How to use pen and paper tasks to aid tremor diagnosis in the clinic. Pract Neurol. 2017;17(6):456–463.
17. Höglinger GU, Respondek G, Stamelou M, et al. Clinical diagnosis of progressive supranuclear palsy: The movement disorder society criteria. Mov Disord. 2017 Jun;32(6):853–864.
18. Rittman T, Coyle-Gilchrist IT, Rowe JB. Managing cognition in progressive supranuclear palsy. Neurodegener Dis Manag. 2016 Dec;6(6):499–508.
19. Grimes DA, Lang AE, Bergeron CB. Dementia as the most common presentation of cortical-basal ganglionic degeneration. Neurology. 1999 Dec 10;53(9):1969–1974.
20. Shir D, Pham NTT, Botha H, et al. Clinicoradiologic and neuropathologic evaluation of corticobasal syndrome. Neurology. 2023 Jul 18;101(3):e289–e299.
21. Day GS, Lim TS, Hassenstab J, et al. Differentiating cognitive impairment due to corticobasal degeneration and Alzheimer disease. Neurology. 2017 Mar 28;88(13):1273–1281.
22. Cui Y, Cao S, Li F, et al. Prevalence and clinical characteristics of dementia and cognitive impairment in multiple system atrophy: A systematic review and meta-analysis. J Parkinsons Dis. 2022;12(8):2383–2395.
23. Cubo E, Shannon KM, Tracy D, et al. Effect of donepezil on motor and cognitive function in Huntington disease. Neurology. 2006;67(7):1268–1271.
24. Jay JA, Kumar V, Garrels E, et al. Management of neuropsychiatric disturbances in Huntington's disease: A literature review and case report. Prim Care Companion CNS Disord. 2023 Jan 26;25(1).
25. Hoche F, Guell X, Vangel MG, et al. The cerebellar cognitive affective/Schmahmann syndrome scale. Brain. 2018 Jan 1;141(1):248–270.
26. Manto M, Mariën P. Schmahmann's syndrome—identification of the third cornerstone of clinical ataxiology. Cerebellum Ataxias. 2015;2:2.
27. Nishida Y, Hizume M, Fumimura Y, et al. Cerebellar cognitive affective syndrome improved by donepezil. Intern Med. 2019 Apr 1;58(7):1003–1006.
28. Toniolo S, Pisotta I, Manto M. Editorial: The role of the cerebellum in dementia and neurodegenerative diseases. Front Neurosci. 2023;17:1229624.
29. Lu K, Nicholas JM, Pertzov Y, et al. Dissociable effects of APOE ε4 and β-amyloid pathology on visual working memory. Nature Aging. 2021 2021/11/01;1(11):1002–1009.

30. Austad SN, Hoffman JM. Is antagonistic pleiotropy ubiquitous in aging biology? Evolution, Medicine, and Public Health. 2018;2018(1):287–294.
31. Andrade-Guerrero J, Santiago-Balmaseda A, Jeronimo-Aguilar P, et al. Alzheimer's disease: An updated overview of its genetics. Int J Mol Sci. 2023 Feb 13;24(4).
32. Liu P-P, Xie Y, Meng X-Y, et al. History and progress of hypotheses and clinical trials for Alzheimer's disease. Signal transduction and targeted therapy. 2019 2019/08/23;4(1):29.
33. David MCB, Giovane MD, Liu KY, et al. Cognitive and neuropsychiatric effects of noradrenergic treatment in Alzheimer's disease: Systematic review and meta-analysis. Journal Neurol Neurosurg Psychiatry. 2022;93(10):1080–1090.
34. Koch G, Motta C, Bonnì S, et al. Effect of rotigotine vs placebo on cognitive functions among patients with mild to moderate Alzheimer disease: A randomized clinical trial. JAMA Network Open. 2020;3(7):e2010372–e2010372.
35. La AL, Walsh CM, Neylan TC, et al. Long-term trazodone use and cognition: A potential therapeutic role for slow-wave sleep enhancers. J Alzheimers Dis. 2019;67(3):911–921.
36. Barker MS, Gottesman RT, Manoochehri M, et al. Proposed research criteria for prodromal behavioural variant frontotemporal dementia. Brain. 2022 Apr 29;145(3):1079–1097.
37. Breton A, Casey D, Arnaoutoglou NA. Cognitive tests for the detection of mild cognitive impairment (MCI), the prodromal stage of dementia: Meta-analysis of diagnostic accuracy studies. Int J Geriatr Psychiatry. 2019 Feb;34(2):233–242.
38. Hackett K, Krikorian R, Giovannetti T, et al. Utility of the NIH Toolbox for assessment of prodromal Alzheimer's disease and dementia. Alzheimers Dement (Amst). 2018;10:764–772.
39. Pertzov Y, Miller TD, Gorgoraptis N, et al. Binding deficits in memory following medial temporal lobe damage in patients with voltage-gated potassium channel complex antibody-associated limbic encephalitis. Brain. 2013;136(8):2474–2485.
40. Nianogo RA, Rosenwohl-Mack A, Yaffe K, et al. Risk factors associated with Alzheimer disease and related dementias by sex and race and ethnicity in the US. JAMA Neurol. 2022 Jun 1;79(6):584–591.
41. Knight R, Khondoker M, Magill N, et al. A systematic review and meta-analysis of the effectiveness of acetylcholinesterase inhibitors and memantine in treating the cognitive symptoms of dementia. Dement Geriatr Cogn Disord. 2018;45(3–4):131–151.
42. Xu H, Garcia-Ptacek S, Jönsson L, et al. Long-term effects of cholinesterase inhibitors on cognitive decline and mortality. Neurology. 2021;96(17):e2220–e2230.
43. Cummings J. Meaningful benefit and minimal clinically important difference (MCID) in Alzheimer's disease: Open peer commentary. Alzheimers Dement (NY). 2023 Jul-Sep;9(3):e12411.
44. Rodríguez-Calero MA, Blanco-Mavillard I, Morales-Asencio JM, et al. Defining risk factors associated with difficult peripheral venous cannulation: A systematic review and meta-analysis. Heart & Lung. 2020 2020/05/01/;49(3):273–286.
45. Sims JR, Zimmer JA, Evans CD, et al. Donanemab in early symptomatic Alzheimer disease: The TRAILBLAZER-ALZ 2 randomized clinical trial. JAMA. 2023.
46. van Dyck CH, Swanson CJ, Aisen P, et al. Lecanemab in early Alzheimer's disease. N Engl J Med. 2022;388(1):9–21.
47. Budd Haeberlein S, Aisen PS, Barkhof F, et al. Two randomized phase 3 studies of aducanumab in early Alzheimer's disease. J Prev Alzheimers Dis. 2022;9(2):197–210.
48. Beisteiner R, Matt E, Fan C, et al. Transcranial pulse stimulation with ultrasound in Alzheimer's disease: A new navigated focal brain therapy. Adv Sci (Weinh). 2020 Feb;7(3):1902583.
49. Luo Y, Sun Y, Tian X, et al. Deep brain stimulation for Alzheimer's disease: Stimulation parameters and potential mechanisms of action [review]. Front Aging Neurosci. 2021 March;11;13.
50. Kavirajan H, Schneider LS. Efficacy and adverse effects of cholinesterase inhibitors and memantine in vascular dementia: A meta-analysis of randomised controlled trials. Lancet Neurol. 2007 Sep;6(9):782–792.
51. Taylor JP, McKeith IG, Burn DJ, et al. New evidence on the management of Lewy body dementia. Lancet Neurol. 2020 Feb;19(2):157–169.
52. Scales K, Zimmerman S, Miller SJ. Evidence-based nonpharmacological practices to address behavioral and psychological symptoms of dementia. Gerontologist. 2018 Jan 18;58(suppl_1):S88–102.
53. Dudas R, Malouf R, McCleery J, et al. Antidepressants for treating depression in dementia. Cochrane Database Syst Rev. 2018 Aug 31;8(8):Cd003944.
54. Porsteinsson AP, Drye LT, Pollock BG, et al. Effect of citalopram on agitation in Alzheimer disease: The CitAD randomized clinical trial. JAMA. 2014 Feb 19;311(7):682–691.
55. Murphy K, Khan A, Bachu A, et al. Treatment of behavioral and psychological symptoms of dementia using transcranial magnetic stimulation: A systematic review. Int Psychogeriatr. 2023 Feb;20:1–12.

Chapter 3

Delirium

Definition and description

The concept of delirium dates back to antiquity. The etymology of the term originates from the Latin 'delirare' 'to go out of the furrow', i.e., to be derailed, to be going off course, or to be deranged[1]. The initial descriptions date back 2,000 years when Hippocrates described it. Since then there have been repeated attempts at defining this syndrome. The core features of delirium include altered consciousness, global disturbance of cognition, fluctuating course, and perceptual abnormalities. The onset is usually rapid with evidence of an underlying physical cause. Common pathophysiological mechanisms suggested to explain delirium include cerebral metabolic insufficiency, activation of inflammatory pathways, changes in neurotransmitter functioning, and ultimately changes in functional neuronal network connectivity[2].

Core clinical features of delirium

- Acute onset
- Fluctuating course
- Inattention
- Disorganized thinking
- Altered level of consciousness
- Cognitive deficits
- Perceptual disturbances
- Psychomotor disturbance
- Altered sleep/wake cycle
- Emotional disturbances

Typical picture in practice

The onset of delirium is acute and the impairment of consciousness characteristically fluctuates, with deterioration in the evening when environmental stimulation is lowered. *Alertness* or arousal to the surrounding environment can either be lowered or increased. Characteristically, in delirium, the alertness fluctuates between falsely increased alertness and a lowered awareness of the surroundings. Other forms of impairment in consciousness, such as impaired attention and difficulty in estimating the passage of time, can also be seen. The patient can appear to be distractible and may be unable to perform classical tests of concentration such as serial sevens where the patient counts backwards in sevens from 100, spelling the word 'WORLD' backward, or saying the months of the year or days of the week backward. The interpretation of these assessments should take into account the patient's age and educational background.

- The disturbance of *sleep/wake cycle* is also part of the classical presentation of delirium. The patient usually presents with daytime drowsiness and insomnia at night. Excessive dreaming with persistence of the experience into wakefulness is also common.
- *Speech* and *thinking* are abnormal and the rate of speech is either slowed or speeded up. The capacity to make judgements and to grasp abstract concepts also becomes impaired. Thought processes can appear more incoherent and disorganized as the illness progresses. The patient appears to be unable to differentiate between their own thought processes and their external world and can, at times, present as increasingly preoccupied with their inner thoughts and experiences with very little awareness of their surroundings.
- Disturbance of *memory* is also an important feature. Short-term, immediate, and working memory are commonly affected but long-term memories can also be disturbed. The most common presentation is disorientation in time and place with disorientation in time occurring in the milder stage and then progressing on to disorientation in place. A failure to track time and the intermittent nature of some of the deficits can sometimes result in jumbled up memories of past and present which may at times result in false recall.

- Several screening tools exist to identify delirium, including the 4AT rapid clinical test for delirium and the Confusion Assessment Method (CAM). Examples of more detailed assessment scales include the Delirium Rating Scale Revised (DRS-R-98), Memorial Delirium Assessment Scale (MDAS), and the Confusion Assessment Method–Severity (CAM-S).

Further reading

Adamis D, Treloar A, Martin FC, et al. A brief review of the history of delirium as a mental disorder. Hist Psychiatry. 2007 Dec;18(72 Pt 4):459–469.

Wilson JE, Mart MF, Cunningham C, et al. Delirium. Nat Rev Dis Primers. 2020 Nov 12;6(1):90.

Activity levels in delirium

Disturbance of psychomotor *behaviour* is also common. Classically, the patient fluctuates between a lowered state of psychomotor activity and little response to external environment, although inner experiences such as hallucinations or delusions may be present, and the other extreme of psychomotor behaviour presenting as agitation or purposeless behaviour such as groping or picking, which may be associated with complex stereotyped movements. Rarely, psychomotor agitation results in mimicking of a work pattern, sometimes described as occupational delirium.

More recently, the two fluctuating forms of psychomotor disturbance have been described as hyper- and hypoactive delirium:

In hyperactive delirium the patient has heightened arousal and can react to surrounding stimuli with verbally and physically aggressive and threatening behaviour. They usually appear restless and wandersome and may pull repeatedly at clothing—a phenomenon described as 'carphologia' (*Gk.* 'to gather twigs'). Other abnormal hand movements include plucking at the air, known as floccillation[3]. Abnormalities of *perception* such as visual, auditory, or tactile hallucinations are also common in hyperactive delirium. Other disturbances such as abnormal perception of size of visually perceived objects (micropsia and macropsia) or auditory stimuli (hypo- or hyperacusis) have also been described. Illusions (misinterpretation of external stimuli), usually in visual form, are common along with hallucinations (perceptions without objective stimuli). The most common form of hallucination in delirium is visual and may present in many forms, from simple forms such as flashes of light to fully formed scenes of people and animals. 'Lilliputian' hallucinations occur when patients see tiny animals or people.

- The hypoactive type of delirium is much less obvious as patients are withdrawn and do not react to their abnormal perceptual phenomena, which are easily detectable if an effort is made to recognize them. The hypoactive form of delirium is more common but can be easily missed and the patient classically presents as being drowsy, not interested in their environment, and eating and drinking poorly. If spoken to, speech is usually incoherent and they find it difficult to understand questions.

Further reading

Holt R, Teale EA, Mulley GP, et al. A prospective observational study to investigate the association between abnormal hand movements and delirium in hospitalised older people. Age Ageing. 2014;44(1):42–45.

Diagnostic criteria for delirium

Both the ICD and DSM systems require a disturbance in orientation and attention developing over a short time period. Other features may include acute impairments in other cognitive domains (including perceptual distortions, illusions, hallucinations, delusions, and loss of recent memories), psychomotor disturbance (hyper- and hypoactivity), sleep/wake cycle disturbance, and emotional disturbance (e.g. depression, anxiety or fear, irritability, euphoria, apathy, or wondering perplexity). These diagnostic criteria are of real practical use—for example, helping a bewildered clinician in a busy hospital environment to reassure themselves that they are correct in identifying this diagnosis.

- A disturbance of attention, orientation, and awareness developing within a short period of time (e.g. within hours or days), typically presenting as significant confusion or global neurocognitive impairment with transient symptoms that may fluctuate depending on the underlying causal condition or aetiology.
- The disturbance represents a change from the individual's baseline functioning.
- Delirium may be caused by the direct physiological effects of a medical condition, by the direct physiological effects of a substance or medication, including withdrawal, or by multiple or unknown aetiological factors.
- The symptoms are not better accounted for by a pre-existing or evolving neurocognitive disorder (i.e. amnestic disorder, mild neurocognitive disorder, or dementia) or by another mental disorder (e.g., schizophrenia or other primary psychotic disorder, a mood disorder, post-traumatic stress disorder, a dissociative disorder). The symptoms are not better accounted for by a typical syndrome of substance intoxication or substance withdrawal for a substance or medication that is known to be present, although delirium can occur as a complication of intoxication or withdrawal states.

Source: data from the International Classification of Diseases, Eleventh Revision (ICD-11); World Health Organization (WHO) 2019/2021 https://icd.who.int/browse11.

Case example of delirium

An acutely disturbed 70-year-old in a care home

You receive a referral marked 'URGENT' from a local general practice. It states that a 70-year-old gentleman who has been a resident at a care home for the last few years has suddenly become 'aggressive' towards the staff. The routine physical examination is not suggestive of an acute physical illness and his blood results and MSU are normal. He has been prescribed some promethazine 25 mg up to 3 times a day but this is not helping to calm him down. He is known to have hypertension, ischaemic heart disease, and TIAs but has been stable on medication.

On your visit to the care home, the staff, who have known the patient for some years, inform you that for the last 3 days the patient has not been sleeping at night, is wandering in the corridors, and getting into the bedrooms of other residents in the middle of the night. He has been physically aggressive towards members of staff on a couple of occasions when they tried to persuade him to go back to his room. During the daytime, he has been noted to be drowsy, not interested in eating and drinking, and sitting quietly in front of the television in the lounge all day.

You try to interview the patient but he appears very drowsy and disinterested in the conversation. He finds it difficult to keep his eyes open, tries to respond to some of your questions but it is difficult to make sense of what he is saying. Despite repeated attempts, you are unable to do a formal mental state examination or test his cognitive function.

Looking at the list of his previous and current medication, you notice that there have been no major changes apart from a recent stoppage of his regular dose of laxative (lactulose) 2 weeks ago, following a brief episode of diarrhoea. On enquiring from the staff about the patient's bowel habits, you learn that he has been constipated since the lactulose was stopped recently.

You do a PR examination to find that the rectum is full of hard faeces. You ring the GP practice nurse to enquire if she would be able to give the patient an enema and restart him on his regular dose of lactulose.

You ring up the care home after the weekend to enquire about the patient's condition and are told that he had a huge bowel movement after the enema and his behaviour has gradually improved over the last 2 days. The staff have, however, been giving him promethazine 3 times a day, which makes him drowsy during the daytime. You suggest omitting the morning and afternoon dose of promethazine and keeping the night-time dose for a few more days until the sleep cycle comes back to normal.

Common causes of delirium

Predisposing factors in delirium

- Old age (over 65 years).
- Male sex.
- Visual impairment.
- Presence of dementia.
- Severity of dementia.
- Depression.
- Functional dependence.
- Immobility.
- Hip fracture.
- Dehydration.
- Alcohol dependence.
- Physical frailty.
- Deafness.
- Malnutrition.
- Catheterization.

Precipitating factors in delirium

- Lower respiratory tract infections.
- Urinary tract infections.
- Constipation.
- Electrolyte imbalance.
- Orthopaedic surgery.
- Cardiac surgery.
- Pain and sleep deprivation.

Drugs that may cause delirium

- Drugs with high anticholinergic activity:
    - Cimetidine
    - Prednisolone
    - Theophylline
    - Tricyclic antidepressants (e.g. amitriptyline)
    - Digoxin
    - Nifedipine
    - Antipsychotics (e.g. chlorpromazine)
    - Furosemide
    - Ranitidine
    - Isosorbide dinitrate
    - Warfarin
    - Codeine
    - Captopril
- Other drugs associated with delirium:
    - Benzodiazepines
    - Narcotics
    - Antiparkinsonian agents (e.g. L-dopa)
    - NSAIDs

- Over-the-counter drugs associated with delirium:
  - Diphenhydramine (e.g. Benylin)
  - Chlorpheniramine (e.g. Piriton)
  - Promethazine (e.g. Phenergan, Night Nurse)
  - Antidiarrhoea drugs (containing atropine, e.g. lomotil)
  - Irritable bowel syndrome drugs containing hyoscine (e.g. Buscopan)

(Source: data from Burns A, Gallagley A, Byrne J. Delirium. J Neurol Neurosurg Psychiat. 2004;75:362–367; Young J, Inouye SK. Delrium in older people. BMJ. 2007;34:842–846.)

Distinguishing delirium from other mental illnesses: 1, Dementia

Although delirium can occur in people suffering from any form of psychiatric illness, distinguishing delirium from dementia and psychosis are the two common clinical dilemmas.

Delirium and dementia overlap

In older people, distinguishing delirium from dementia can present as a clinical challenge as the two conditions have overlapping aetiology and clinical features (Table 3.1). Patients with dementia are known to be at an increased risk of developing delirium, and vice versa. Out of the three common types of dementia, distinguishing delirium from DLB can be most difficult as both illnesses present with prominent visual hallucinations and a fluctuating course.

The safest course of action in cases where there may be an overlap between the two illnesses is to consider delirium as the primary diagnosis and manage accordingly.

Table 3.1 Comparing delirium and dementia

Feature	Delirium	Dementia
Development	Sudden	Slow
Duration	Days to weeks	Months to years
Presence of other disorders or physical problems	Almost always present, may be a severe illness, drug use or withdrawal, or a problem with metabolism	Possibly none
Variation at night	Almost always worse	Often worse
Attention	Greatly impaired	Maintained until late stages
Level of consciousness	Fluctuates from lethargy to agitation	Normal until late stages
Orientation to surroundings	Varies	Impaired
Use of language	Slow, often incoherent and inappropriate	Sometimes difficulty finding the right word
Memory	Jumbled and confused	Deficient, especially for recent events
Mental function	Lost, variably and unpredictably	Lost, relatively consistently for all functions
Cause	Usually an acute illness or drugs. In older people, usually infection, dehydration, or drugs	Usually AD, VaD, or DLB
Need for treatment	Urgent medical attention	Non-urgent attention

Distinguishing delirium from other mental illnesses: 2, Psychosis

Delirium and an acute psychotic illness can have a number of common presenting features and Table 3.2 should be helpful in distinguishing the two from each other. From a management point of view, however, as with dementia, all cases suspected of an overlap of delirium and psychosis should be managed with delirium being the primary diagnosis.

Table 3.2 Distinguishing dementia from psychosis

Clinical features of delirium	Common signs of delirium	Common signs of psychosis due to a psychiatric disorder
Orientation	Confusion about current time, date, place, or identity	Usually aware of time, date, place, and identity
Attention	Difficulty paying attention	Retention of ability to pay attention
Short-term memory	Loss of recent memory	Retention of recent memory
Abstract thinking	Inability to think logically	Inability to think logically
Concentration	Inability to perform simple calculations	Retention of ability to calculate
Delusions	Preoccupations commonly inconsistent	Preoccupations often fixed and consistent
Hallucinations	Hallucinations (if any) mostly visual or involving touch	Hallucinations (if any) mostly auditory
Physiology	Fever or other signs of infection	No infection signs History of previous psychiatric disturbances
Drug use/abuse	May have history of alcohol misuse	Alcohol misuse rare

Coronavirus (COVID) and old age psychiatry

The COVID pandemic had profound impacts on the lives of older people around the world, from the isolation felt by those who could not be visited, to the hurricane of lethal infections that tore through many care homes for older people in the early stages of the pandemic. The long-term outcomes, including long COVID syndromes with psychiatric symptoms, and the effects on long-term risk of dementia, are not yet clear.

Psychiatric symptoms during acute COVID illness

Acute COVID infection is dominated by familiar symptoms including shortness of breath, cough, anosmia, and fever. Inevitably, any acute respiratory illness leading to anoxia in older people will cause many cases of delirium. Directly acute neuropsychiatric syndromes due to central nervous system (CNS) involvement of COVID-19 virus are probably rare.

Psychiatric syndromes after acute COVID

Accumulating data show that the risk of common psychiatric syndromes (depression and anxiety) is definitely increased after COVID infection, but the risk is probably transitory. For more serious conditions including psychotic illness and dementia, there is increased risk which persists for at least 2 years[1].

COVID and risk of neurological syndromes

About a third of patients with acute COVID will develop a neurological symptom—in many cases the symptom (fatigue, myalgia, anosmia) may be of non-neurological mechanism. In the period after acute COVID the risk of stroke is probably 5–6-fold higher than that after other viruses like influenza[2]. Specifically, neuropsychiatric syndromes, i.e. encephalopathy with ataxia, delirium, and seizure, have been reported but are probably rare.

COVID and mood

Most evidence suggests a real but transitory increased risk of depression after infection. Clinical experience has shown that isolation for older people caused profound emotional effects, not just transitory. Careful study of the effects of isolation has clearly shown that shielding (the practice of actively isolating older people to minimize social encounters) independently increased the risk of depression, and reduced older people's quality of life[3]. In any future pandemics, it is likely that mental health risks can be actively weighed in deciding social policy.

Case vignette 1

An 84-year-old man was admitted to acute hospital with difficulty breathing. His temperature was 38.5°C and he needed oxygen by nasal prongs but not continuous positive air pressure (CPAP) or Intensive Care Unit (ICU) support. He received dexamethasone. He spent five days in hospital before going home with a limited care package. His abbreviated mental test (AMT) score in hospital varied from 6/10 to 9/10. Nursing staff say he is forgetful and family say he is below his cognitive baseline. He is referred to a memory clinic for follow-up.

Case vignette 2

A 79-year-old woman has a history of breast cancer and recently had surgery and chemotherapy. She is widowed and lives alone, independently. Her three children live 20–40 kilometres away. They organize online food deliveries and repeat prescriptions are dropped off to her home. A daughter phones daily. She appears increasingly withdrawn and apathetic. She begins not to answer the phone, worrying the family. She confides in a grandson that she feels there is little to live for. After shielding ends, she is reluctant to return to old hobbies and will only go out with a family member present, reporting anxiety also. Her family feel that COVID caused this—she had no confirmed case, though did report an episode consistent with upper respiratory tract infection 3 months into her shielding.

References

1 Taquet M, Gillett B, Zhu L, Mendel J, Camplisson I, Dercon D, et al. Lancet Psychiat. 2022; 9(10):815–827.

2 Misra S, Kolappa K, Prasad M, RadhaKrishnan D, Thakur K, Solomon T, et al. Neurology. 2021 7 Dec;97(23):e2269–e2281.

3 Di Gessa G, Price D. B J Psych. 2022; 221(4):637–643.

Managing the delirious patient in general hospital—principles

Delirium is a common condition seen in hospital patients. Its problems and incidence are particularly high in surgical in-patients, such as those undergoing cardiothoracic and orthopaedic procedures, in-patients undergoing cataract surgery, or those in ICUs. High rates of delirium have also been reported in patients admitted to cancer units and those having dialysis due to renal failure.

Management

Delirium is a medical emergency with a high morbidity and mortality risk. Any patient suspected of having delirium requires prompt attention, while recent evidence suggests that the most successful approach to delirium should also concentrate on its prevention.

Strategies for delirium prevention

Identification of high-risk patients for developing delirium, such as those with hip fractures, can lead to significant reductions in the incidence, severity, and duration of delirium. Evidence for delirium prevention strategies comes mostly from non-randomized trials; it is estimated that 30–40% of cases may be preventable. The following strategies tailored according to the needs/risk factors of the individual patient can be used in delirium prevention and all involve an assertive approach across all high-risk patients:

- Orientating communication.
- Therapeutic activities.
- Early mobilization and walking.
- Maintaining nutrition and hydration.
- Adaptive equipment for vision and hearing impairment.
- Adequate pain management.
- Avoiding sedation.
- Use of non-pharmacological intervention for sleep disturbance.
- Early discharge.
- Home rehabilitation services.

Identification of underlying cause and precipitating factors

- In practice, the commonest causes are infections, metabolic and fluid imbalance, cerebral hypoxia, pain, sensory deprivation, urinary retention, faecal impaction and polypharmacy.
- A detailed history and examination along with review of the results of investigation provides a guide to understanding the cause. A raised white blood count or specific symptom (such as a fever) may indicate an infection process. Asymptomatic bacteriuria is common in older people and a positive MSU does not necessarily mean that it is the only cause of the symptoms.
- Dehydration, cerebral hypoxia caused by congestive cardiac failure, and unrecognized severe pain should be ruled out in all in-patients with delirium.

Maintaining behaviours

Hospital in-patients, especially with hyperactive delirium, can be at risk of falls, non-compliance with medication/interventions leading to delayed/poor recovery, exposure to extremes of temperature, harm to self and others. Agitation, aggression, and wandering are the most common behavioural disturbances requiring pharmacological and non-pharmacological interventions.

Preventing complications and supporting functional needs

A number of strategies including adequate pain control, withdrawal of unnecessary drugs, supportive care including management of hypoxia, hydration, and nutrition along with mobilization, participation in ward activities such as physiotherapy, and minimizing time spent lying in bed are likely to contribute to early resolution of delirium.

Management of delirium in a general hospital—key tips

- **Hospital admission**: identify high-risk cases, taking into account the possible predisposing and precipitating factors.
- **Use a standardized delirium assessment tool**: tools such as the CAM can aid diagnosis.
- **Perform a baseline mental and cognitive state examination**: observe for changes in mental and cognitive state.
- **Observe changes in cognitive/mental state**: identify if the change is of acute onset or an aggravation of pre-existing illness such as dementia or psychosis.
- **For all acute changes in mental/cognitive state:** evaluate for the possibility of delirium using the diagnostic criteria. Try to rule out dementia, depression, and acute psychosis. Get specialist advice at this stage and don't wait for symptoms to become more complicated. Treat all acute changes/disturbance in mental and cognitive state as delirium.
- **Identify and eliminate predisposing and precipitating factors**: this process would include obtaining history for alcohol/drug abuse and benzodiazepine use, monitoring vital signs, detailed physical and neurological examination, and laboratory tests which may include the following: MSU, FBC, B_{12} and folic levels, thyroid function test (TFT), LFT, blood gas levels, ECG, lumbar puncture, and neuroimaging.
- **Review medications**: try to eliminate or alter all unnecessary medications that might contribute to delirium.
- **Prevent complications**: this would include procedures such as protecting the airways, preventing aspiration pneumonias, maintaining adequate hydration and nutritional support, skin care, mobilization, and prevention of deep-vein thrombosis.
- **Managing agitated patients actively**: only use pharmacological interventions for severely agitated patients, and as a general rule start with a low dose and titrate until the desired behavioural control is achieved. Try to use oral medication and use the parenteral route if oral medication is not possible.
- **Use non-pharmacological intervention**: environmental alterations and aids to reduce sensory deprivation such as eyeglasses and hearing aids are the most important.

Tips for clinicians using the Confusion Assessment Method

These apply when using other delirium assessment scales.[1]

Acute onset and fluctuating course: You will need to ask a carer or family member to know this. The key here is change from baseline, and rapid fluctuation, i.e. several times in the same day, not just in the last week or month.

1 Source: data from: Inouye SK (2003), *The Confusion Assessment Method (CAM): Training manual and coding guide*. Boston, MA, Yale University School of Medicine; Young J, Inouye SK (2007). BMJ, 2007;34:842–846.

Inattention: Can they focus on conversation (with you) or on a task (e.g. giving the days of the week backward).

Disorganized thinking: Do they seem to you to ramble, go off track on to irrelevant topics?

Altered level of consciousness: Level of consciousness can range from comatose, through normal, to excessive (hypervigilance).

Managing the delirious patient in a care home

Delirium in care homes is common and a number of factors including old age, medical comorbidity, polypharmacy, sensory impairments, and dementia can put care home residents at higher risk of developing delirium.

History and background information

- A careful history of the events leading up to the start of illness should be taken. The staff at the care home that have known the patient for some time are the best people to provide this information. Identification of the onset (acute or chronic), pattern of deterioration, sleep/wake cycle, food and fluid intake, changes in bowel habits, sensory deficits (deafness, cataracts, loss of spectacles and hearing aids) should be considered.
- A careful history of signs of acute infections, such as urinary tract infections, upper and lower respiratory tract infections, and skin infections should be taken.
- A detailed review of the patient's current list of medications, recent changes of dose/addition of new medications with possible deliriogenic effects should be made.
- Personal distress caused by pain and its causes (varying from arthritis to metastatic cancer) should be taken into account. Chronic or acute on chronic constipation is a common cause of delirium and should always be considered in patients at care homes.

Past medical history

- Ischaemic heart disease and cardiovascular disease (CVD) along with metabolic disorders should be considered. An aggravation of an already existing chronic physical disease such as renal or hepatic failure could have precipitated delirium.
- Past history of psychiatric illnesses such as schizophrenia, bipolar affective disorder, depression, and anxiety is important in the assessment as they could complicate the clinical picture or the presentation might be due to a recurrence of a psychotic illness.

Mental state and cognitive examination

- There is no short cut to a detailed mental state and cognitive examination. As the diagnosis of delirium rests on the clinical skill of the physician, special emphasis should be laid on the patient's appearance, signs of agitation, perceptual abnormalities, and cognitive disturbances, including reduced attention and concentration and shifting attention.
- Use of diagnostic instruments can sometimes be helpful, and nursing staff can be trained to administer them. The Confusion Assessment Method (see section *Management of delirium in a general hospital—key tips*, this chapter) is a widely known instrument which is easy to administer, and is available in long and short versions. The shorter version has only 4 questions and takes minutes to complete.

Investigations/management

- Routine investigations such as MSU, FBC, LFT, U&E levels, lipid profile, and TFT should be carried out urgently. An ECG (although not always practically possible to carry out in care homes) could be helpful in ruling out a recent cardiac event—recent developments in ambulatory care make such tests potentially easier to arrange.
- Management should involve a combination of environmental and pharmacological interventions.
- The staff should be made aware of the provisional diagnosis and environmental modifications required for the particular patient such as encouraging wakefulness during the day and replacement of spectacles or hearing aid, administration and timing of medication to control severely disturbed behaviours, and strategies to prevent escalation of agitation by using medication at the earliest signs of behavioural disturbance. The pharmacological interventions may also include a course of antibiotics for an ongoing infection, laxatives for relieving constipation, and painkillers for adequate pain control.
- Other management strategies might also include involving professionals from other disciplines in the patient's care, such as podiatrists to tackle painful/infected in-growing toenails, physiotherapists to provide exercise plans for arthritis, referrals to pain clinics for adequate pain relief with medications, skin patches, or acupuncture.

Follow-up

- It is essential that the treatment plan for delirious patients should include follow-up due to the high morbidity and mortality, especially in patients with underlying dementia.
- The follow-up should include a review of the results of investigations, effectiveness of the management plan (both pharmacological and non-pharmacological), and examining other interventions such as seeking specialist advice or hospital admission if the symptoms are not subsiding or are aggravating. This is especially important in a care home environment where patients can be more vulnerable than hospital inpatients and a contingency plan with the care home staff should be discussed, such as calling out emergency ambulance services if the condition deteriorates. Direct communication with the specialist/hospital staff by the referring doctor can be helpful in avoiding unnecessary delays by repeating investigations/assessment by the hospital staff.

Pharmacological management of delirium

Pharmacological management should be planned according to the symptomatology of an individual patient and would generally aim at control of symptoms (delusions and hallucinations), improving the sleep/wake cycle, and controlling agitation and aggression.

It is useful to formulate a management plan and clearly identify the symptoms/behaviours to be targeted with pharmacological intervention before prescribing medication.

The following steps are useful in making a pharmacological intervention plan:

- A careful analysis of the risks and benefits of drug treatment.
- A review of the current list of medications and consideration of stopping the possible 'deliriogenic' drugs may be useful.
- Making staff aware of early symptoms that could potentially escalate to cause behavioural disturbance can result in reduced use of medication.
- Oral administration of medication should be the preferred route of administration unless it is contraindicated or not possible due to lack of insight or behavioural disturbance.
- Administering medication parenterally (intramuscular or intravenous) can be challenging for the staff and a clear plan about the possible use of physical restraint can be useful. This is especially important if the staff are not trained to use restraint and may require the help of psychiatric nursing staff.
- Antipsychotics (typical and atypical) are the mainstay of treatment in patients with psychotic or hyperactive presentations.
- Amongst typical antipsychotics, haloperidol is usually the drug of choice. It has been found to be effective in a number of RCTs. It has a short duration of action and can cause extra-pyramidal side effects and prolongation of the QT interval. It is usually safe in comorbid medical conditions but should be avoided in alcohol withdrawal syndrome and hepatic failure. The usual dose recommended for the elderly is 0.5–1 mg twice a day orally with additional doses every 4–6 h if required. In severely disturbed and aggressive patients it can be given intramuscularly (0.5–1 mg) and repeated after 30–60 min until the behaviour is controlled. It can also be used intravenously (IV) in extremes of behavioural disturbance but should not be used IV as a routine because of its short duration of action.
- Among atypical antipsychotics, risperidone (0.5 mg twice daily), olanzapine (2.5–5 mg once daily), and quetiapine (25 mg twice a day) can be used. Risperidone and olanzapine have been associated with increased risk of cerebrovascular events and mortality in patients with dementia. These drugs have an advantage of having slightly less risk of causing extra-pyramidal side-effects compared with haloperidol. They do, however, prolong the QT interval.
- Benzodiazepines may be particularly helpful where the delirium is caused by withdrawal of alcohol or sedatives. Benzodiazepines with rapid onset and short duration of action, such as lorazepam, are preferred and can be given orally or in extreme emergencies, IV. Lorazepam (0.5–1 mg) with additional doses every 4–6 h can be used

as a second-line agent in treating all forms of delirium and as a first-line agent in treating delirium due to sedative and alcohol withdrawal, Parkinson's disease, and neuroleptic malignant syndrome. It is known to sometimes cause over-sedation, respiratory depression, and sometimes, paradoxical excitation.

- Some other drugs such as trazodone, a tricyclic-related antidepressant, in doses of 25–150 mg orally at bedtime may be useful in treating delirious patients with a disturbed sleep/wake cycle and night-time disturbance. More recently, some reports about the possible use of cholinesterase inhibitors in treating and preventing delirium have emerged but there have been no convincing controlled trials demonstrating their efficacy, and some evidence that they may worsen prognosis in ICU patients with delirium.

Non-pharmacological management of delirium

The non-pharmacological approach is equally, if not more, important than pharmacological interventions and should be an integral part of the management plan, tailored according to the needs of an individual patient.

Environmental modification

This aims at creating a calm and comfortable environment for the disturbed patient, taking into consideration the following:

- Noise control.
- Use of orientating influences, such as calendars, clocks, and familiar objects from home.
- Regular communication and reassurance by the staff and limiting room and staff changes.
- Involving family members in supportive care.
- Avoiding procedures such as venepuncture and catheterization at night-time to allow the patient to have uninterrupted periods of sleep.
- Encouraging normal sleep/wake cycles by dimming the lights and providing a calm environment at bed-time and encouraging wakefulness and mobility during the day.
- Encouraging early mobilization, especially after orthopaedic surgical procedures, by involving physiotherapists and podiatrist to provide a structured routine of physical activity during the waking hours.

Sufferers' experiences of delirium

Reports suggest that patients may recall their experience of delirium more vividly than expected from the profound disturbances in consciousness and awareness. These reports suggest that up to 80% of patients with delirium can recall their experiences (often in great detail) and a similarity between the experience of delirium and the recall of dreams has been noted. These observations emphasize the importance of non-pharmacological interventions such as patient listening, reassurance, and orientation techniques. Many such reports recall the experience of helplessness and terror common among patients with delirium; bear this in mind when organizing care.

Further reading

Burns A, Gallagley A, Byrne J. J Neurol Neurosurg Psychiat. 2004;75:362–367.
Fairburn AF (2002). Delirium—An overview. In *Principles and practice of geriatric psychiatry*, 2nd edn (ed. JRM Copeland, MT Abou-Saleh, and DG Blazer). Chichester, John Wiley and Sons, pp. 179–182.
Inouye SK. Delirium in older persons. N Engl J Med. 2006;354:1157–1165.
Crammer JL. Subjective experience of a confusional state. Br J Psychiatry. 2002 Jan; 180:72–75.
Young J, Inouye SK. Delrium in older people. BMJ. 2007;34:842–846.

References

1. Adamis D, Treloar A, Martin FC, et al. A brief review of the history of delirium as a mental disorder. Hist Psychiatry. 2007 Dec;18(72 Pt 4):459–469.
2. Wilson JE, Mart MF, Cunningham C, et al. Delirium. Nat Rev Dis Primers. 2020 Nov 12;6(1):90.
3. Holt R, Teale EA, Mulley GP, et al. A prospective observational study to investigate the association between abnormal hand movements and delirium in hospitalised older people. Age Ageing. 2014;44(1):42–45.

Chapter 4

Mania and depression

Mania and depression—an overview

- Late-life depression (LLD) describes a depression with late onset, chronic course, and poorer response to antidepressant medications. The vascular depression hypothesis suggests a disease process which involves small vessel cerebrovascular insults, limbic hyperactivity, and endothelial dysfunction. A constellation of cognitive features suggestive of a medial frontal lobe syndrome have been associated with LLD, encapsulated in the term 'depressive executive dysfunction' (DED). Working memory, verbal fluency, and response inhibition can all be affected. These findings have suggested that insults to key frontolimbic networks are responsible[1].
- Several characteristic presentations may also be encountered among older patients, including severe psychomotor retardation, pseudodementia, and hypochondriacal states. Psychotic symptoms should be probed for closely in severe cases. Suicidal thoughts or plans should be explored, and a risk management plan instituted if need be.
- In addition to LLD, manic-depressive (bipolar) illness can present in older adults in various forms. When assessing older patients presenting with mania for the first time, acute organic causes may be responsible, so-called secondary mania. A thorough history, laboratory testing, and neuroimaging may be warranted, depending on the context.
- However, primary bipolar illness in older adults is possible. Late-onset bipolar (LOBP) may present in patients who have had a tendency to mood changes throughout their life, experiencing subsyndromal symptoms but never reaching clinical significance previously[2]. Rather than experiencing a mood episode during their childhood or adolescence, these patients may have experienced subsyndromal symptoms ('mood temperaments'). A careful history, including family history, is essential. In contrast to LLD, the course is episodic and recurrent, mixed, and manic symptoms may be present, and monoaminergic drugs may worsen the patient's symptoms or can cause a 'switch'.

Differential diagnosis

History

[illegible]

[illegible] differentials

- [illegible]
- Neurodegenerative disorders (including Alzheimer's disease (AD), [illegible] disease (PD), [illegible] (FTD), [illegible] Huntington's disease, and [illegible]).
- Multiple sclerosis.
- Traumatic brain injury (TBI).
- Endocrine conditions, including [illegible]
- [illegible]
- [illegible]
- Substance or medication induced mood disorder. [illegible]
- Sleep disorders.

[illegible]

[illegible]

- [illegible]
- [illegible]
- [illegible]
- [illegible]
- [illegible]
- [illegible]
- [illegible]

Differential diagnosis

History

For patients with prior diagnoses of mood disorders, these should be explored, including which management strategies worked in the past. For new-onset cases, delirium and important organic causes should be ruled out, depending on the presentation. The full medical and drug history should be sought, and is also useful in planning medication choices and avoiding drug interactions, if indicated after the assessment. The diagnosis can be reached by characterizing the patient's symptoms, course of illness, relevant family history, and response to any treatments. The patient's functioning and general psychosocial status can be assessed by taking a brief personal and social history. Psychotic symptoms and suicidality should be probed for.

Acute organic differentials

- Acute post-stroke syndromes, right-sided lesions probably associated with mania, left-sided probably with depression.
- Neurodegenerative disease, including Alzheimer's disease (AD), Parkinson's disease (PD), fronto-temporal dementias (FTD), phenocopy FTD, Huntington's disease, and basal ganglia calcification.
- Multiple sclerosis
- Traumatic brain injury (TBI)
- Endocrine conditions, including Cushing's disease, syndrome of inappropriate antidiuretic hormone secretion (SIADH).
- Tumour.
- Infection, including HIV.
- Substance or medication induced mood disorder. Typical examples include steroids, alpha-interferon, and anti-parkinsonian medication.
- Sleep disorders.

Note: this list is not exhaustive, a wide range of general medical conditions can lead to depressive or manic symptomatology.

Primary manic and depressive syndromes

- Late-life depression (LLD). Often patients present with a chronic, worsening, moderate to severe depression associated with vascular disease ('vascular depression'). Depression executive dysfunction (DED) is common[3].
- Primary late-onset bipolar illness (LOBP).
- Patient with a prior history of a bipolar diagnosis experiencing recurrence of symptoms ('graduates'), also known as early-onset bipolar illness (EOBP). See Ghaemi et al. (2022) for the full range of presentations[4].
- Several specifiers exist in current diagnostic manuals, including whether psychotic or catatonic symptoms are present and the presence of mixed features.
- Melancholic features refers to a triad of psychomotor retardation, anhedonia and lack of mood reactivity.
- Other specifiers in the DSM-5 include anxious distress, atypical features, or seasonal pattern.
- 'Other' or 'Unspecified' categories exist to capture variations which do not fit exactly into the above groups.

Investigations

Routine bloods may be helpful, and neuroimaging depending on the clinical presentation, e.g. to rule out relevant organic causes. Baseline liver and renal function tests can inform pharmacotherapy options.

Possible investigations dependent upon the patient's symptoms:

- Bedside investigations including temperature and urine dipstick
- FBC
- U&E
- LFT
- CRP
- B12, folate, vitamin D
- Other electrolytes including calcium, magnesium, phosphate
- TFT
- Drug and alcohol screen
- Endocrine tests for Cushing's or Addison's disease
- Neuroimaging (e.g. MRI), especially looking at the prefrontal cortex, cingulate cortex, and limbic structures.

Biomarkers

There are several hypotheses about the underlying mechanisms of LLD, but none of the putative biomarkers are used routinely in clinic (see section on *Late-Life Depression*). Additionally, there are currently no routine biomarkers in use for identifying OABP or for monitoring progression or treatment response. Tomasik and colleagues reported on a possible new biomarker test which could distinguish between bipolar (BP) and other depressive diagnoses[5]. The test consists of a dried blood spot (DBS) metabolomic signature (see Fig. 4.1). Interestingly, the results indicated that sphingolipids, in particular ceramides, may be involved in the pathophysiology of BP. Sphingolipids have been implicated in neuronal cellular pathophysiology, including in lipidomic studies[6,7]. However, this has not been validated in older adults, in whom metabolic signatures may differ. Other future biomarkers may be based on neuroimaging, e.g. use of T1-weighted MRI measures of accelerated ageing for disease staging[8].

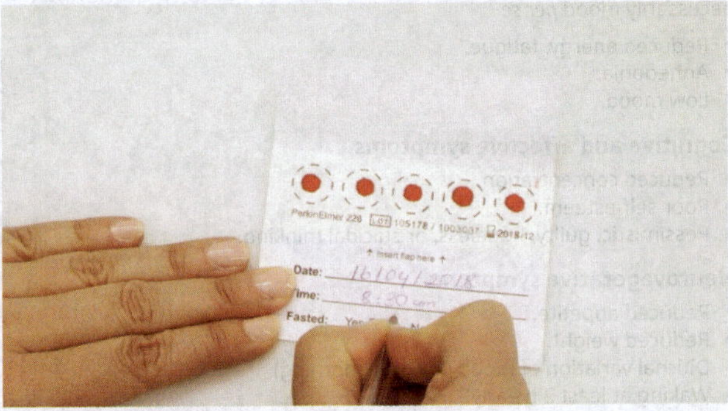

Fig. 4.1 Dried blood spot (DBS) test.

Reproduced courtesy of Professor Sabine Bahn, University of Cambridge.

Symptoms and diagnosis

Diagnosis is based on careful history taking together with observation of core abnormalities of mental state. Symptoms alone are insufficient—diagnostic validators are required to make a diagnosis[9]. These are gathered in the history-taking process and from investigations. These include the course of illness, family history, and response to any treatments.

Depressive symptoms are very common; the identification of a depressive episode is based on agreed thresholds for clusters of symptoms occurring together. These symptoms are recognized in DSM-5 and ICD-11 and are the same for older and younger patients. A depressive illness is recognized when symptoms persist for several weeks and interfere with function. Individual episodes should usually last 2 weeks or more and are classified as mild, moderate, or severe. Repeated studies have shown that significant depression, at a level considered worth treating by expert clinicians, is persistent, causes distress, and is associated with poor psychiatric, physical, and social outcomes.

In bipolar illness, recurrence of mood episodes is key rather than polarity *per se*. Clues to the diagnosis include depressive episodes with mixed features, poor response to SSRIs in the past, including manic switching or phenomena such as antidepressant-associated chronic irritable dysphoria (ACID). Medical comorbidities are associated with bipolar disorder, especially migraine[10]. Bipolar type I requires manic episodes somewhere in the history, whereas bipolar type II requires hypomanic episodes. The distinction is severity and duration. In both bipolar I and II, there are also depressive episodes. Manic episodes consist of a period of elevated or irritable mood and increased energy, along with several other symptoms (3 or more, see below). If the episode lasts a week or is particularly severe, then it is classified as manic. If lasting 4–7 days and less severe, then this is considered hypomanic. However, manic symptoms lasting for shorter than this time period are also relevant[11]. Recent evidence has found that the bipolar I versus II dichotomy is less clear in older adults[12].

Core depressive symptoms

The phenomenology of depressive states is about psychomotor slowing, not necessarily mood *per se*.

- Reduced energy, fatigue.
- Anhedonia.
- Low mood.

Cognitive and affective symptoms

- Reduced concentration.
- Poor self-esteem.
- Pessimistic, guilty, hopeless, or suicidal thinking.

Neurovegetative symptoms

- Reduced appetite.
- Reduced weight.
- Diurnal variation of mood (lower in morning).
- Waking at least 2 h early.
- Insomnia.
- Agitation or psychomotor retardation.

Classic presentation of mania

Phenomenologically is psychomotoric activation and an increase in goal directed activity. There is lack of insight.

- Elevated, expansive, or irritable mood.
- The 'DIGFAST' mnemonic can be used to remember other symptoms:
  - *D*istractibility
  - *I*mpulsivity
  - *G*randiosity
  - *F*light of ideas
  - *A*ctivity increased
  - *S*leep reduced or circadian disturbance
  - *T*alkativeness

Mixed features

The 'DAIA' symptoms are associated with greater severity[13]:

- *D*istractibility
- *A*nxiety
- *I*rritability
- *A*gitation

Psychotic and severe symptoms

- Delusions, especially mood congruent delusions of a nihilistic type, failure, extreme guilt, deserving of punishment, poverty, hypochondriacal (e.g. has cancer).
- Hallucinations especially voices commenting on an individual's supposed failure, commands to self-harm, or olfactory hallucinations (e.g. of rotting flesh).
- Suicidal thoughts and plans.
- Melancholia: psychomotor retardation, anhedonia, and lack of mood reactivity.
- Stupor; patient is mute, unresponsive, and immobile but awake. This may be associated with risk of death from dehydration.

Presentations more likely in older than younger patients

- Agitation.
- Psychomotor retardation.
- Hypochondriasis/somatization (physical symptoms predominate for patient).
- Histrionic behaviour (e.g. throwing oneself on the floor).
- Dangerously poor food/fluid intake.
- Pseudodementia (depression presenting with significant cognitive impairment).

Late-life depression

Vascular depression

Biological factors which may cause depressive illness have been very extensively researched in younger people—especially genetics, neuroendocrine studies, and functional imaging. Key findings in depression include enhanced genetic risk, changes in key neural circuits mediating manic or depressive symptoms, and alterations in functional connectivity. 'Vascular depression' (VaDep) is a term essentially describing the hypothesis that there is a distinct disease in older age characterized by a chronic depressive course and caused by small vessel cerebrovascular insults. Inflammatory processes have also been implicated. It has led to a search for confirmatory evidence and a focus on interventions for vascular disease as a secondary intervention for some people with depression. Clinically, compared to younger adults, features such as anhedonia, psychomotor retardation, and lack of insight are more common[1]. Cognitive symptoms are often present, e.g., depression executive dysfunction (DED, see below).

MRI-defined VaDep is characterized by a range of cerebrovascular disease presentations and white matter hyperintensities (WMHs)[14]. This leads to disruption in frontal-subcortical circuits which regulate reward, salience, and cognition [1,14]. Summary of findings:

- Depression is commoner in post-stroke patients.
- MRI WMHs are more common in depressed than non-depressed older people.
- WMHs are more common in late-onset than early-onset depression.
- WMHs predict a poorer response to treatment of depression.
- Neuroimaging shows limbic hyperactivity and changes in cerebral blood flow.
- Endothelial dysfunction.

Vigorous treatment of depressive symptoms and of vascular conditions like diabetes, atrial fibrillation, and hypertension remain common-sense interventions.

Depression executive dysfunction (DED)

- Cognitive symptoms in LLD often include slowed processing speed, reduced executive functioning, and apathy[12]. Working memory, verbal fluency, and response inhibition may be affected[3]. There may also be lack of insight with mild neurovegetative symptoms[1]. This constellation of findings is called the depression executive dysfunction (DED) syndrome and has been associated with WMHs, functional connectivity disturbances, and poor response to SSRIs [3].

Psychological and social factors in later life

Depressive states in response to psychosocial stressors are common. Old age is a time of considerable readjustment; to frailty, to loss of family/partners, to changes in accommodation. Several factors have well-known effects on mood which are important both in considering individual cases and in establishing high-risk populations. In these instances, management should include a focus on interventions which address the major life changes which the individual has to navigate, including psychotherapeutic approaches. These include:

- Bereavement.
- Isolation/loneliness.
- Disability.
- Life events including moving house, financial, relationship events.
- Social role changes, e.g. ceasing caring role as childminder.
- Caring role, especially for person with dementia.
- Residence—residential home versus own home.
- Personality type/psychological style.

Further reading

Alexopoulos GS. Mechanisms and treatment of late-life depression. Transl Psychiatry. 2019;;9(1):188. [1]

Older age bipolar illness

Classic mania, with overactivity, self-important ideas, and euphoric mood, may present for the first time in older age; graduation of patients with bipolar affective disorder from younger life is more common. When mania is associated with a clear organic illness, the term 'secondary mania' may be used. Medications used in treating mania, especially lithium, have increased side-effect and interaction potential in older people.

Definition

'Older age bipolar illness' (OABP) is a heterogeneous term which encompasses both new cases which develop in later life, late-onset bipolar (LOBP) and 'graduate' patients with younger age of onset, early-onset bipolar (EOBP). An International Society for Bipolar Disorders task force suggested an age of onset of at least 50 defined LOBP, but the exact age varies between studies[2]. Five to 10% of patients experience their first manic episode in later life, with 25% of the bipolar population over the age of 60[3]. LOBP cases may be secondary to an organic cause, or can be primary presentations. General medical comorbidity and cognitive impairment is common in OABP.

Clinical characteristics and epidemiology

Patients continue to suffer from symptom recurrence into later life, and mood episodes have not been shown either to worsen or abate due to changes with age[15,16]. However, differences have been found in symptom severity and nature. The Global Aging & Geriatric Experiments in Bipolar Disorder (GAGE-BD) database is an international effort to pool together data to characterize patient trajectories in OABP. The investigators analysed data from 1,374 patients (mean age = 60) across 19 cohorts to examine how symptoms varied over time[17]. Overall, they found that the severity of manic and depressive symptoms was attenuated by time. However, this may represent a 'survivor' cohort of patients diagnosed with EOBP (mean age of onset = 31). Symptom mixity appears to be common in OABD. An analysis from the GAGE-BD database of approximately 800 patients showed that 70% of patients experienced symptoms with mixed features[18]. A further analysis found that there was little distinction between BP I and II in OABP[12].

In addition to general medical comorbidity, cognitive changes are characteristic of OABP. A meta analysis of 328 euthymic patients diagnosed with OABP found deficits, with a large effect size, in verbal learning and delayed memory when compared to controls[19]. Other areas of worse performance included working memory, immediate memory, processing speed, cognitive flexibility, attention, and executive function[19]. Language and visuoconstructive cognition were found to be unaffected.

Aetiology

Primary LOBP may be distinct from EOBP, but there is limited data characterizing this group[20,21]. Some patients may have experienced unipolar depressive episodes previously and then been diagnosed with LOBP once they presented with mania or hypomania. Another possibility is patients with underlying mood temperaments or subsyndromal symptoms who present with more severe symptoms later in life. The ageing process, increased cerebrovascular burden, and a raised incidence of sleep/wake disorders have all been postulated as factors involved in pathogenesis.

A systematic review and meta-analysis of neuropathological changes in BP at all ages found decreased cortical thickness in the subgenual anterior cingulate cortex and reduced neuronal density in the amygdala and prefrontal cortex[22]. Neurobiological findings include disrupted endocrine function, dopamine function, calcium signalling, and circadian rhythms[23]. Functional neuroimaging studies suggest lateralized disruption of limbic circuits in mania, consisting of left hemispheric limbic hyperactivity with hypoactivity of the right ventromedial and ventrodorsal prefrontal cortex[24].

There is a relative paucity of data in OABP specifically, though. Villa and colleagues[25] examined cortical thickness and grey matter volume in OABP. They found widespread reduction in cortical grey matter and also in the amygdala, thalamus, and hippocampus. Those with later onset, in this study defined as ≥ 25 y, had a distinct phenotype, defined by reductions in cortical thickness (insular, temporal, parietal, occipital, parahippocampal) and reductions in the striatum, hippocampus, and thalamus[12]. Of note, patients diagnosed with OABP who had attempted suicide were found to have reduced cortical thickness in the dorsolateral prefrontal cortex (DLPFC)[12].

The link between OABP and neurodegenerative disorders is complex. Cognitive deficits have been observed in OABP, but the underlying pathology is not neurodegenerative. Many of these changes also affect memory. However, sometimes mood symptoms can be prodromal of neurocognitive disorder and there is an increased risk of dementia in patients diagnosed with OABP. FTD can be mistaken for BP, due to disinhibition and manic symptoms, presumably due to pathology affecting the same neural circuits. Interestingly, lithium's neuroprotective properties have led to studies examining its effects in amnestic MCI (aMCI). In an RCT of 61 patients diagnosed with aMCI randomized either to subtherapeutic lithium (0.25–0.5 mEq/L) or placebo, Forlenza and colleagues found a trend towards slower progression in the lithium group.

Further reading

Long-term lithium treatment in older adults with MCI

Forlenza OV, Radanovic M, Talib LL, Gattaz WF. Clinical and biological effects of long-term lithium treatment in older adults with amnestic mild cognitive impairment: randomised clinical trial. Br J Psychiatry. 2019 Nov;215(5):668–674.

A helpful overview in distinguishing clinical presentations in EOBP, with descriptions of symptoms, course and treatment response:

Ghaemi SN, Angst J, Vohringer PA, et al. Clinical research diagnostic criteria for bipolar illness (CRDC-BP): rationale and validity. Int J Bipolar Disord. 2022 Oct 13;10(1):23.

Special presentations of depression in older people: 1, Pseudodementia

Case example

A 76-year-old woman is referred to psychiatric services with a 6-month history of poor self-care, 'confusion', poor eating, recent incontinence of urine, and poor performance on primary care screening tool for cognitive impairment. For some months she has also been low in mood, lacked confidence, and feels hopeless about the future. At clinic, she scores only 16/30 on MoCA, often answering 'I don't know'. Her family expresses concern that she has dementia, and say she has 'just given up'. CT brain shows some mild periventricular small vessel disease, and atrophy appropriate for age with no lobar predominance. Blood tests show no abnormality.

'Pseudodementia' is a term used for any non-organic cause of dementia which can resolve with resolution of the underlying problem. The term usually refers to depressive pseudodementia. The patient is likely to show poor self-care, lack of concentration, and may appear very forgetful. On testing, deficits are worst on attentional tasks, for example, concentration (e.g. serial sevens or 'WORLD' backward), retrieval of short-term memories, but less likely in 'cortical' tasks, e.g. apraxia/dysphasia. The latter deficits would strongly suggest organic dementia. In the 1980s pseudodementia was felt to be a common misdiagnosis. More recent work has shown that the majority of older people who present with serious cognitive deficits while depressed do not recover full cognitive function, while those who do are at increased risk of subsequent dementia.

Management points

- Clear history—which came first, depression or cognitive impairment?
- In mental state examination are there clear features of depression—sad appearance, hopelessness, psychomotor retardation, or agitation?
- On cognitive testing, does the patient do worse on attentional tasks like spelling WORLD backwards, digit reading, or serial sevens?
- Are there a lot of 'I don't know' answers?
- Is memory performance better with cueing (e.g. hinting at the answer)?
- If depressed, treat with therapeutic course of antidepressant, e.g. SSRI for 6–8 weeks, and augment/change antidepressants if no response.
- Do not make final diagnosis of dementia until a vigorous course of treatment has been achieved. Use term 'possible dementia' while matter is still in doubt.
- May be appropriate to do dementia screen in the interim (blood screen/neuroimaging) in anticipation of persistent cognitive deficits.

Special presentations of depression in older people: 2, Hypochondriasis (somatic symptom disorder)

Case example

An 84-year-old man has a history of arthritis and congestive cardiac failure. He has been attending much more frequently than normal in primary care. He reports a headache and worries that he may have a brain tumour. He reports poor sleep, weight loss, and 'I just can't enjoy anything because of this'. His wife died 6 months previously.

Hypochondriasis means an unjustified morbid fear of illness. A closely related term is 'somatization', which refers to presentations to see a clinician with unexplained physical symptoms which cannot be explained by organic factors but don't respond to reassurance. Depressive illness should be suspected in all such cases. Fear of cancer is particularly likely in older people with severe depression. Preoccupation may be total, leading to relentless pursuit of hospital tests and admission. The hypochondriacal ideas may reach delusional intensity. Such ideas will usually resolve when underlying depression is treated.

Management points

- Clarify the history clearly, especially evidence for depressive illness.
- It is often useful to examine the patient physically to reassure them, establish credibility of the clinician, and avoid surprises during treatment.
- Medically qualified clinicians may find uncertainty about symptoms easier to handle than other professionals, e.g. nurses.
- New investigation may still be needed; a parallel approach of investigating while treating underlying causes of hypochondriasis may in fact be appropriate.
- Consider pharmacotherapy (e.g. SSRI) and if delusional, add low-dose antipsychotic, e.g. 2.5–5.0 mg olanzapine daily.
- Set strict appointments (i.e. regular and not in response to health concerns of patient) and call a halt to further investigations.
- Use judgement if new symptoms arise; older people have much higher incidence of new physical illness.

Special presentations of depression in older people: 3, Severe retardation

Case example

A 79-year-old woman is referred with a history over several weeks of low mood, reduced appetite and weight, not going out, and poor communication. Primary care ask for an urgent psychiatric opinion as she has in the last 3 days stopped communicating, is incontinent, eats barely any food, and is drinking only 300 ml of fluids per day. On assessment, she is clinically dehydrated. She rocks back and forth on a chair and makes little eye contact. She constantly whispers 'it's no good, it's no good'. She refuses all offers of help from nurses, social services, and family.

Presentations of depression with severe retardation are more frequent in older people. Other features found are likely to include suicidal ideation, psychotic symptoms especially nihilistic, hypochondriacal, or guilty delusions, agitation (inner sense of restlessness associated with motor overactivity), and poor food and fluid intake. In older people, progression to malnutrition, and particularly to dehydration, is particularly likely and makes prompt assessment essential. These clinical features predict a favourable response to ECT, which may need to be given against the will of the patient.

Management points

- Urgent assessment is required.
- Assess nutrition and hydration status of patient—look for dry lips and tongue, low blood pressure, weak rapid pulse, change in skin turgor, diminished consciousness.
- Admission to hospital usually required, if necessary compulsorily.
- Baseline investigations in hospital should include those needed to assess anaesthetic fitness—physical examination, U&E, FBC, ECG, chest X-ray.
- Arrange fluid balance chart and parenteral rehydration if needed.
- Assess suicidal ideas in deciding observation required on ward—suicide risk may increase as retardation lessens but depressive ideation remains.
- Acute choice of treatment likely to be between ECT or a combination of antidepressant with antipsychotic.
- Particular concern is needed if the patient shows signs of catatonic stupor—mute, unresponsive and akinetic but still alert. Patients with this presentation are likely to need detention under the Mental Health Act and use of high-dose benzodiazepines or ECT, as well as IV fluids. They may require admission to a general hospital at first.

Assessment scales

Practical use of assessment scales

Rating scales are useful in identifying and quantifying disease severity, some of which are designed specifically for geriatric populations (e.g. the Geriatric Depression Scale). The Young Mania Rating Scale (YMRS) is used to assess manic symptoms. Scales such as the Rapid Mood Screener (RMS) can identify OABP. The Temperament Scale of Memphis, Pisa, Paris and San Diego (TEMPS) can be used to probe for underlying mood temperaments.

After treatment has started, severity scales can be used to estimate response. A 50% or greater reduction in severity indicates reliable response, 25–50% indicates partial response, and < 25% indicates no response. In geriatric clinical trials, there is often a requirement that patients included also score above the cutoff for mild cognitive impairment on a cognition scale (e.g. the MoCA), which may also be warranted in some clinical scenarios. Cognitive impairment should not in itself exclude a trial of treatment for depression—treatment may also improve cognition.

Geriatric Depression Scale

The GDS is probably the best known and most widely used instrument for detection of depression among older people and is particularly appropriate for screening[1]. It takes about 5 min (15-item version) and can be self- or rater-administered. The original version has 30 items and tends to avoid physical/somatic items which will be endorsed by people with physical illness. It has been developed as a 15-, 10-, and even 4-item version. All have been shown to be valid and reliable, though reliability is lowered in more severe dementia. The 15-item version is now widely used including in primary care.

Montgomery and Asberg Depression Rating Scale

The MADRS is a well-validated scale needing an interviewer to spend 20 minutes with the patient[2]. It rates severity of symptoms in 10 important areas. This scale was designed to be sensitive to change and is especially useful in establishing the effects of treatment. Psychological items dominate, making it suitable for use in older people.

Young Mania Rating Scale

Widely used rating scale for manic symptoms, the YMRS comprises 11 questions, 4 of which are scored out of 8, and 7 out of 4. Takes about 15–30 minutes to administer. Recommended by the GAGE-BD group for manic symptoms in OABP.

Patient Health Questionnaire 9

The PHQ-9 is a nine-item self-report scale for depressive symptoms[3]. Probably less well validated among older people than other measures. Easy to use and has demonstrated sensitivity to change.

Quick Inventory of Depressive Symptomatology

QIDS is a self assessment scale of 16 items which has become more popular recently in clinical practice and trial settings. A longer Inventory of

Depressive Symptomatology (IDS) exists. Both QIDS and IDS have a clinician rated and patient rated version.

Temperament Scale of Memphis, Pisa, Paris and San Diego

TEMPS is a questionnaire which identifies cyclothymic, hyperthymic, or dysthymic temperament. Patient-rated, true and false question stems.

Rapid Mood Screener

RMS is a short, pragmatic 6-item screening tool for bipolar disorder which performs comparably to longer alternatives.

National Institute of Health (NIH) Toolbox Emotion Battery

A range of touchscreen tests of affect, well-being, and stress. Demonstrating an increase in positive subscales is increasingly being used in clinical trials as a primary endpoint in conjunction with demonstrating a reduction in absolute depression ratings on traditional assessment measures.

Centre for Epidemiological Studies—Depression Scale

This 20-item scale (CES-D) is self-administered and takes about 5 min to complete[4]. Originally developed for general populations, it is more popular for use with older people. Validity against traditional instruments is established, though caution is advised with visually or cognitively impaired people.

Hamilton Depression Rating Scale

HDRS is one of the best-known depression rating scales and one of the commonest scales used in trials of antidepressant medication[5]. It takes about 20 min for an interviewer to administer and establishes the severity of symptoms in 17 domains. The time required and the number of physical symptoms may limit its practical usefulness in older clinical populations.

Further reading

Lavin P, Rej S, Olagunju AT, et al. Essential data dimensions for prospective international data collection in older age bipolar disorder (OABD): Recommendations from the GAGE-BD group. Bipolar Disorders. 2023;25(7):554–563.[26]

References

1. Yesavage J, Brink T, Rose T, Lum O, Adey M, Leirer O. Development and validation of a geriatric depression screening scale: A preliminary report. J Psychiat Res. 1983;17:37–49.
2. Montgomery S, Asberg M. A new depression scale designed to be sensitive to change. Br J Psychiatr. 1979;134: 382–389.
3. Kroenke K, Spitzer RC, Williams JBW. The PHQ-9. J Gen Intern Med. 2001;16:606–613.
4. Radloff L, Teri L. Use of the Centre for Epidemiological Studies Depression Scale with older adults. Clin Gerontol. 1986;5:119–137.
5. Hamilton M. A rating scale for depression. J Neurol Neurosurg Psychiatr. 1960; 23:56–62.

GDS-15

This depression rating scale is particularly suited to older people as it avoids confounding by physical illness, i.e. focuses on core psychological symptoms of depression rather than somatic symptoms such as appetite or weight loss[1]. Though an effective screening tool, it is not diagnostic so does not replace clinical judgement. Undertake the test orally (can be given as a self-rated sheet—omit bold print for this). Ask the patient to reply indicating how they have felt over the past week. Get a clear yes or no reply. Bold answers score one point.

1. Are you basically satisfied with your life? Yes/**No**
2. Have you dropped many of your activities and interests? **Yes**/No
3. Do you feel happy most of the time? Yes/**No**
4. Do you prefer to stay at home rather than going out and doing new things? **Yes**/No
5. Do you feel that life is empty? **Yes**/No
6. Do you often get bored? **Yes**/No
7. Are you in good spirits most of the time? Yes/**No**
8. Are you afraid that something bad is going to happen to you? **Yes**/No
9. Do you feel helpless? **Yes**/No
10. Do you feel that you have more problems with memory than most? **Yes**/No
11. Do you think it is wonderful to be alive? Yes/**No**
12. Do you feel pretty worthless the way you are now? **Yes**/No
13. Do you feel full of energy? Yes/**No**
14. Do you feel that your situation is hopeless? **Yes**/No
15. Do you think that most people are better off than you are? **Yes**/No

Scoring

0–4	No depression
5–8	Mild depression
10+	Severe depression

Reference

1. Sheikh JL, Yesavage JA. Geriatric Depression Scale (GDS): recent evidence and development of shorter versions. Clin Gerontol. 1986;5:819–820.

Management of acute mania

General approach

- Assess risk levels—aggression, self-neglect, overspending, legal problems, deterioration, stress to carers.
- Manic symptoms describe a general psychomotor activation. Patients may be markedly distractible, anxious, or irritable rather than euphoric in mood.
- Decide where to treat, including involuntary admission if necessary.
- Ensure adequate hydration.
- Baseline blood tests to include U&E, FBC, and TFT.
- If mild illness, use a mood stabilizer alone—lithium, carbamazepine, or valproic acid.
- If more severe initiate antipsychotic treatment adjunctively in the short term, e.g. haloperidol 5–10 mg/day in divided doses or olanzapine 10 mg/day.
- Consider using parenteral treatment if non-compliant (e.g. intramuscular haloperidol or olanzapine).
- For long-term prophylaxis, initiate a mood stabilizer.
- Maintain observation in in-patients until absconsion/non-compliance risks are acceptable.
- Observe closely for emergence of depressive symptoms during treatment and particularly for suicidal ideas.

Outcome of mania

- The outcome of manic episodes among older people is the same as younger people—with treatment, full recovery within 1–2 months is usual. Issues thereafter relate to the particular importance of compliance with mood-stabilizing medication and the general need to monitor patients at high risk of further illness. Cycling directly into severe depression carries particular risks for older people, while in all age groups, when treating for bipolar depression, watch for the risk of precipitating a manic episode.

Case example

An 85-year-old patient with a history of recurrent depression has recently changed: her family doctor refers her to specialist services. Her husband is exhausted and reports she has slept poorly, been spending more money, giving money away to local youths, and has been irritable. She denies there is anything wrong. At interview, she is irritable, voluble, and somewhat euphoric. Her speech is pressured. She has no grandiose ideas but is certain that there is nothing wrong. Cognitively, she scores only 21 on MoCA, losing points on concentration tasks in particular. She agrees to admission, believing it is for medical reasons. U&E is normal and she is initiated on lithium and olanzapine. Her sleep improves rapidly and mania subsides. After 2 months, back home, she remains psychiatrically well but is gaining weight. She comes off olanzapine but remains on lithium. She has 3-monthly blood tests. Her urea oscillates between 6.0 and 8.0, and creatinine between 90 and 130. Her lithium level varies between 0.4 and 0.6 mmol/L. She develops a slight tremor of the upper limbs. Eventually she moves to a care home after her husband dies, and a district nurse keeps regular lithium testing going.

Drugs for mania

Lithium

- Lithium has been known since the late 1940s to have antimanic action. It took nearly three decades to be widely used as clinicians were concerned by its toxicity which had been demonstrated in the 1940s when lithium salts were used as an alternative to sodium chloride in the diet of people with hypertension. Lithium is antimanic, has mood-stabilizing effects for people with bipolar illness, and also is used to augment the effects of antidepressants. It has waned in popularity, but is considered a disease-modifying agent in bipolar illness and is the best choice for maintenance treatment if clinically appropriate. At normal levels (usually clinicians aim for blood levels of 0.4–0.8 mmol/L 12 h post-dose), lithium can cause tremor, a metallic taste, some diuresis, and can cause hypothyroidism. Used long term, lithium can cause declining renal function in some patients, probably due to renal parenchymal damage.
- It has an unknown mode of action. Lithium is neuroprotective and may work through multiple mechanisms including neurotrophic factors, genes affecting circadian rhythms, GSK3 inhibition, and AMPA receptor downregulation[27,28]. One hypothesis is that lithium exerts its effects by a mechanism known as homeostatic synaptic scaling, in which the strength of a neuron's synapses are modulated or 'tuned'[29]. In one study, lithium was found to elicit synaptic downscaling which may ameliorate excess glutamatergic neurotransmission[27].
- Lithium is usually given as a carbonate once at night. At normal levels (blood concentration 0.4–0.8 mmol/L) it can cause tremor, metallic taste, diuresis, hypothyroidism, and may worsen renal function. At toxic levels (over 1.5 mmol/L) it can cause diarrhoea and vomiting, coarse tremor, confusion, convulsions, coma, and death. Toxicity is more likely in patients on non-steroidal anti-inflammatory drugs (NSAIDs), thiazide diuretics, and in those dehydrated. It may be more likely in older people, who use these drugs more often. Avoidance of toxicity depends on regular blood tests (3-monthly lithium levels taken around 12 h after usual dose) and counselling about symptoms.

Suggested lithium regime

- Baseline U&E, TFTs, calcium[30].
- 200-400mg nocte of lithium carbonate, depending on renal function.
- Lithium level to be taken 5-7 days later, 12h post dose (in morning).
- Adjust dose to establish level between 0.4 and 0.8 mmol/L.
- Most patients can tolerate a level of 0.9 or 1.0 mmol/L, at least for a period. Repeat lithium level after 1-2 weeks more.
- 3-monthly blood tests—lithium level, TFTs, U&E.

The GERI-BD trial

In the only double-blind RCT in geriatric bipolar disorder, 224 patients were randomized to either lithium or valproate[31]. Adjunctive, open-label risperidone was an option for non-responders. Outcome was measured by YMRS. The authors hypothesized that valproate would be better tolerated, however this was not the case. The authors conclusion was that 'both lithium and divalproex were adequately tolerated and efficacious; lithium was associated with a greater reduction in mania scores over 9 weeks'.

Valproic acid

An anticonvulsant drug which enhances gabaergic inhibition of neurotransmission. It is often given as Depakote (semisodium valproate). It is contraindicated in women of child-bearing age. Valproate has been associated with neurodevelopmental disorders in the children of fathers (of any age) taking it, and requires careful counselling (see further reading below). Valproic acid can cause gastric irritation, weight gain, drowsiness, and blood dyscrasias. Its main problem is the potential for serious hepatic dysfunction—it should not be started without baseline LFTs. Fulminant liver failure is rare, transient increases in LFTs are more common. Doses should start low (250 mg/day of Depakote) and be increased carefully.

Carbamazepine

Carbamazepine blocks voltage-gated sodium channels. Therapeutic window less clear-cut than with lithium. Main problems are likely to be blood dyscrasias (regular FBC recommended though patients should be aware of symptoms), hyponatraemia (probably more common in older people, regular U&E needed), and dose-related dizziness and unsteadiness. Carbamazepine is a liver enzyme inducer; it may decrease the effect of warfarin, some analgesics, and antibiotics. Doses should be started low (100–200 mg/day) and increased in steps of 100–200 mg/day.

Lamotrigine

Lamotrigine is an anticonvulsant which is used primarily for prophylaxis of depressive episodes in bipolar illness and also in rapid cycling (i.e. 4 or more episodes per year). A rare but important side effect is toxic epidermal necrolysis or Stevens–Johnson syndrome. Start with 25–50 mg once daily and titrate up over a period of weeks.

Dopamine receptor blockers

Dopamine receptor blockers (i.e. antipsychotics) undoubtedly have antimanic effects and may work faster than mood stabilizers alone. The antimanic effects are probably due to antidopaminergic action. Dopamine blocking agents can also be used for depressive symptoms in bipolar illness. Higher doses may be needed than for late paraphrenia, especially in acute manic episodes. Older patients with depressive illnesses are at high risk of tardive dyskinesia (TD) and other risks to consider are known cardiovascular/mortality risks in presence of dementia, and weight gain with olanzapine used long term. Quetiapine is a popular choice for presentations across the bipolar spectrum. Newer second-generation antipsychotics (SGAs) are recommended in recent guidelines which have a lower liability for side effects, for example, lurasidone, lumateperone, and cariprazine. Olanzapine-samidorphan (opioid receptor antagonist) combinations have less liability for weight gain[32].

Further reading

Valproate use in men

Medicines and Healthcare products Regulatory Agency, United Kingdom. Valproate use in men: as a precaution, men and their partners should use effective contraception. 2024. https://www.gov.uk/drug-safety-update/valproate-use-in-men-as-a-precaution-men-and-their-partners-should-use-effective-contraception

The GERI-BD trial

Young RC, Mulsant BH, Sajatovic M, et al. GERI-BD: A randomized double-blind controlled trial of lithium and divalproex in the treatment of mania in older patients with bipolar disorder. Am J Psychiatry. 2017 Nov 1;174(11):1086–1093.

Lithium's effects on synaptic plasticity

Kavalali ET, Monteggia LM. Targeting Homeostatic synaptic plasticity for treatment of mood disorders. Neuron. 2020 Jun 3;106(5):715–726.

An overview of regulatory approvals and evidence for new SGAs and formulations

2023–2024 Florida Best Practice Psychotherapeutic Medication Guidelines for Adults (2023). The University of South Florida, Florida Center for Behavioral Health Improvements and Solutions.

Psychological, social, and behavioural treatment of depression

While social interventions such as befriending or social groups are often initiated for older people with depression, psychological treatment is underused. Reasons for this may include lack of provision of services, a perception that older people do less well in psychological therapy (Freud described older people as 'ineducable'), a perception that older people may not want psychological treatment, or a belief that cognitive impairment will interfere with progress in treatment. Though the vast majority of trials of psychological treatment for depression have been among younger adults, it is now clear that psychotherapy is an effective treatment among older people. Cognitive behavioural therapy (CBT), problem-solving therapy (PST), and interpersonal therapy have been utilized in older populations[1]. ENGAGE, a therapy which targets specific cognitive problems, especially reward valency, in older depressed adults, has also shown efficacy and is grounded in neurobiological changes in LLD[1].

In bipolar illness, psychoeducation, advice on setting a good routine, and sleep hygiene are important parts of management. Adjunctive psychotherapies include CBT, family-focused therapy, and interpersonal and social rhythm therapy (IPSRT)[33]. More work is needed in OABP in particular.

Deciding on psychological treatment

- Does the patient have cognitive impairment which would make treatment difficult?
- What is the treatment preference of the patient?
- What psychological treatment is available?
- Group versus individual therapy—depending on availability and preference. Group therapy is a dominant mode of treatment for depression in day hospitals for older people.
- Mode of therapy—the main types of psychological treatment appear equally effective among older people, some may be more targeted to specific problems.

CBT

Based on Aaron Beck's principle that how we think and how we act can influence our mood, rather than the other way round. Therapy typically lasts for 6–20 weekly sessions. Unhelpful beliefs and behaviours are identified and countered cognitively (cognitive therapy) or behaviourally. Both feasible and effective for depression among older people.

Psychodynamic and analytic psychotherapy

Originated from work of Freud a century ago, with several schools such as Jungian or Kleinian approaches. Assumes that psychological distress arises from unresolved unconscious conflicts. Uses techniques including free association and focus on transference (emotional relationship of patient to therapist) to work through major issues. Can last for years. A form of treatment which dominated popular ideas of psychiatry through much of the twentieth century—now rarely available in the United Kingdom on the National Health Service (NHS) but often sought privately. The evidence base for its treatment efficacy for depression in older people is unclear.

Counselling

Term describes a brief therapy where ventilation of distress is encouraged, direct information may be imparted, and problem-solving by the patient is encouraged by the therapist. Counselling is probably appropriate for mild to moderate depression, especially when it has arisen in the context of life stress. It is often provided privately or in primary care.

Social management

Engagement of the patient in social activity to counter absence of positive experiences, regular monitoring of mental state and risks, monitoring of drug dose/side effects, and direct contact with mental health professional are all likely to contribute to patient benefit.

Monoaminergic drugs

Most monoaminergic agents (classically called 'antidepressants') are of about the same efficacy in LLD, and most patients who benefit from an antidepressant recover after 6–8 weeks. LLD, including vascular depression, is less likely to respond to SSRIs, and may require tricyclic antidepressants (TCAs), augmentation, or a neuromodulation approach. First-line antidepressants have broadly similar efficacy, although a network meta analysis suggests that some may be superior in the elderly (vortioxetine, agomelatine, quetiapine, duloxetine, imipramine)[34]. Differences between drugs are largely around side effects. Considerations for older people are medical comorbidity, potential drug interactions, changes in pharmacokinetic handling of the drug, and seriousness of side effects. A particular consideration in recurrent depression is what has worked before—you need a good reason not to use it again if it has worked earlier. In general use lower starting doses in elderly patients, in many cases this is a half dose. Monoamine agonist monotherapy can cause a manic 'switch' if the patient lies on the bipolar spectrum and should be avoided unless a strict strategy to detect and manage the switch is in place.

Selective serotonin reuptake inhibitors

These SSRIs are a class of antidepressants which became widely prescribed during the 1990s and are now the most common antidepressants used at any age. They work by preventing reuptake of the key monoamine neurotransmitter serotonin (5-HT), thus promoting serotoninergic neurotransmission. A number have been shown to work in trials specifically among older people. They have fewer serious side effects than older drugs and are considerably safer in overdose. SSRIs have been recommended in most global guidelines as a first-line drug treatment option for treatment of depression.

SSRI name	*Target daily dose*
Fluoxetine	20 mg
Citalopram	20 mg
Escitalopram	10 mg
Sertraline	100 mg
Paroxetine	20 mg
Fluvoxamine	100–200 mg (divided doses over 100 mg)

Most older people can tolerate initiation on the once-daily full therapeutic dose of fluoxetine, citalopram, escitalopram, and paroxetine. Start sertraline at 50 mg daily. Fluoxetine has a long half-life so can be stopped abruptly. Paroxetine has shortest half-life so must be stopped gradually to avoid withdrawal reactions which may be severe. All may cause early anxiety and gastrointestinal discomfort and all may cause hyponatraemia (stop antidepressant, refer to general medicine if serum Na remains below 125 mmol/L). There is some increased risk of gastrointestinal haemorrhage among older people taking SSRIs.

Serotonin/noradrenaline active drugs

- Mirtazapine (target dose 30–45 mg/day) is a serotonin/noradrenaline active agent which is particularly useful in sleepless patients. Monitoring of FBC may be needed as it may cause blood dyscrasias. Can be combined with venlafaxine.
- Venlafaxine is a serotonin/noradrenaline reuptake inhibitor (SNRI). The target dose is usually 112.5–150 mg/day, though higher doses may be needed for some patients. There is a concern about raised blood pressure at the higher doses and withdrawal can be difficult for some patients.
- Duloxetine (target dose 60 mg/day) also works by preventing reuptake of both serotonin and noradrenaline (SNRI). It is generally well tolerated.

Tricyclic antidepressants

TCAs are a class of drug that led the era of antidepressant prescribing from the 1950s, when imipramine was introduced. These drugs are undoubtedly effective in depression and appear to exert their effect by preventing reuptake of serotonin and noradrenaline into presynaptic nerve endings. They have many other effects including alpha-receptor blockade (causing hypotension), anticholinergic effects (causing dry mouth, urinary retention, constipation), drowsiness, and in higher doses destabilization of the cardiac membrane, making them particularly dangerous in overdose. Equally effective agents with fewer side effects have made new prescriptions less common. Commonly used tricyclic antidepressants include imipramine, amitryptiline, clomipramine, dothiepin, trimipramine, and a more modern tricyclic called lofepramine (target dose 70– 210 mg/day), which has fewer toxic effects. Lofepramine can be useful in patients who are hyponatraemic. In older people, tricyclic antidepressants should be started at low doses (e.g. 25mg/day for amitryptiline, 10 mg/day for clomipramine or imipramine) and built up slowly, warning the patient about likely side effects.

Monoamine oxidase inhibitors

MAOIs comprise a class of drug that was introduced in the 1950s but has fallen out of favour due to potential interaction with certain drugs, e.g. other antidepressants, nasal decongestants, and opiate analgesics, and with tyramine-containing foods, which may precipitate a hypertensive crisis. A newer reversible and selective MAOI, moclobemide, has fewer restrictions on use and is a useful alternative to older MAOIs such as phenelzine and tranylcypromine. This class of drug should only be considered after advice from a psychiatrist.

Multimodal and other drugs

- **Vortioxetine**, a multimodal, serotoninergic medication is efficacious and a systematic review found that it has procognitive effects in elderly depressed patients[35]. Start at 5 mg and increase up to 20 mg if needed.
- **Bupropion** has dopaminergic action, in addition to noradrenergic effects. Start at 150 mg OD with a target of 300 mg.
- **Agomelatine** has activity at MT1/MT2 melatonergic receptors, and also 5-HT2C antagonism. Its melatonergic actions make it different to other drug classes. Agomelatine requires LFT monitoring upon initiation. Start at 25 mg ON, increasing to 50 mg after 2 weeks. Arrange LFTs at 3, 6, 12, and 24 weeks of treatment.

Drug treatment—next-line

In general, expect 60–70% of older people with depression to respond to a full course of an adequate dose of an antidepressant. For those who do not, a change in treatment strategy is needed. This may include a change to a non-drug treatment (e.g. neuromodulation) or psychological treatment (such as CBT).

There are several considerations in difficult to treat depression. It may be that the diagnosis is wrong. Diagnostic possibilities include cognitive impairment or medication induced symptoms. It is worth assessing the patient's cognitive function and reviewing any regular medicines which they take. A significant percentage of patients diagnosed with unipolar depression in fact have been found to experience undetected subsyndromal bipolar symptoms and therefore require a different psychopharmacological approach[36]. In addition to asking about mixed features or an underlying mood temperament, use of a structured bipolar screening tool or mood temperament scale can help to identify bipolar spectrum presentations. Another is that the clinical picture is better explained by personality traits or personality disorder, in which case the patient's case should be reformulated and the treatment plan altered accordingly to focus on relevant psychotherapeutic interventions. Unaddressed, challenging social issues will confound the efficacy of drug treatment in LLD.

Next step pharmacological options include:

- Increase dose.
- Switch class.
- Augment.

Increase dose

Rarely likely to be helpful if a therapeutic dose has been achieved (e.g. already on 20 mg/day of citalopram, fluoxetine, or paroxetine). Increasing to higher doses should only be tried with frequent monitoring for side effects and when there has been at least partial response to initial course of antidepressant.

Switch class

A switch of class of agent is appropriate. A sensible initial strategy is to switch from a first-line SSRI to a noradrenaline/serotonin active agent or multimodal drug. Some patients will respond to a switch to a TCA but the new drug should be started at a lower dose and weekly review to increase dose and review response and side effects is recommended. Switching to an MAOI requires precise washout periods and particular expertise.

Augmentation

Augmentation involves the addition of a new agent to an existing antidepressant drug. The most common agent used in augmentation has been lithium. Small controlled trials support the usefulness of this strategy but lithium interacts with many commonly prescribed drugs among older people, including SSRIs and thiazide diuretics (both increasing the risk of lithium neurotoxicity) so this is another manoeuvre only to be used with specialist review.

Other augmentation strategies include the addition of atypical antipsychotics (especially useful in patients with delusions) or triiodothyronine (T3). Combinations of two antidepressants are sometimes used; this should only be done in specialist hands due to risks of hypertension and severe serotonergic side effects. Augmentation with stimulants is an emerging strategy, which may also be helpful for apathy. A trial of citalopram combined with methylphenidate (5–40 mg) compared with citalopram alone resulted in enhanced efficacy, but both groups had similar improvements in cognitive function[37]. Amphetamines were in fact first marketed for depression, but evidence for treating depressive illnesses is lacking and they are known to have non-specific effects in well individuals,

In the Optimizing Outcomes of Treatment-Resistant Depression in Older Adults (OPTIMUM) trial, Lenze and colleagues (2023) compared augmentation with aripiprazole (2 mg titrated up as required) or bupropion, with a switch to bupropion in elderly patients who had failed to respond to 2 prior antidepressants. The augmentation groups had a roughly similar remission rate (30%) compared to the switch group (approximately 20%). In the next stage of the study, patients who had not responded to either switched to nortriptyline or augmented with lithium. Either strategy produced a roughly 20% remission rate. This illustrates the need for sustained, steady treatment strategies, usually in a specialist clinic, with reasonable chances of eventual recovery, even in highly resistant cases.

How long to treat for?

- Depressive illness usually takes 6–8 weeks for a full recovery.
- Older people are at significant risk of relapse (within 6 months) and recurrence (after 6 months).
- The full dose of antidepressant used to make them well, if tolerated, should be used for at least 6 months, then gradually withdrawn.
- Observe for re-emergence of depression on withdrawal.
- Consider maintenance treatment in any older person you feel is at risk.

Transcranial Magnetic Stimulation

Repetitive transcranial magnetic stimulation (rTMS) is an attractive treatment option because it is non-invasive, does not require an anaesthetic or the work-up required for ECT, and, unlike pharmacological treatments, has relatively few side effects. Unlike ECT, rTMS is also appropriate for a wider range of indications, is not associated with cognitive side effects, and is not restricted to resistant or severe disease states. Furthermore, utilizing neuronavigation, the use of MRI with rTMS, treatment can be targeted to specific regions of interest ('image-guided psychiatry').

In rTMS, electrical pulses are delivered non-invasively to the brain. These pulses are induced by a magnetic field, which in turn is generated by passing an electric current through a coil. The changing magnetic field induces electrical pulses which are delivered to the brain, a demonstration of Faraday's law, a basic law of electromagetism. Modern rTMS machines can deliver multiple pulses in one session, hence the term 'repetitive'. Typically, pulses are delivered through a coil, which is placed over the head to target the desired neuroanatomical regions. TMS machines can deliver these pulses at different frequencies and in different patterns, which are known as treatment protocols. Dose is usually expressed as a percentage of the motor threshold (MT), the energy required to induce contraction of abductor pollicis brevis (thumb). A typical course of TMS would require the patient to attend for a 30–40 minute session, 5 days a week for 4–6 weeks. However, many protocols can be much more rapid and compressed. Several mechanisms of action have been hypothesized, including induction of neuronal plasticity in key networks along with changes in neurotrophic, neuroendocrine, and neurotransmitter systems. In particular, rTMS may modulate fronto-cingulate circuits.

Indications

In general, rTMS is currently used predominantly as a first- or second-line treatment for mood disorders. However, the ability to target specific brain areas means that TMS has been used for a wide range of diseases, with the most evidence for major depressive disorder (MDD), obsessive-compulsive disorder (OCD), anxiety disorders, migraines, and smoking cessation (all of which have at least one regulatory approval globally). Whilst there are less data specifically in older adult populations, a systematic review of the literature suggests that TMS is well tolerated and effective. Treatment protocols may need to be tailored to take into account age-related brain changes, e.g. by increasing total number of pulses or treatment duration to counteract reduced neuronal plasticity. Recent meta-analyses suggest that rTMS may have a beneficial effect on memory in MCI and AD, however, the exact relationship between treatment protocol and cognitive function is not clear currently. Further, meta analysis suggests that rTMS may be effective as an adjunct in Parkinson's disease (PD) for motor and mood symptoms, but again the strength of evidence has not been sufficient to gain a regulatory endorsement. Systematic review data also suggest that rTMS may improve insomnia and sleep symptoms in a neuropsychiatric context, but the risk of bias is high in studies so far.

Contraindications

The main contraindications are relevant to patients who either have metal implants, and therefore could be hurt by the magnetic fields produced by rTMS, and in those who are at risk of seizures. Metallic implants include devices such as cardiac pacemakers and deep brain stimulation electrodes and it is worth keeping in mind that tattoos can contain metallic ink. Seizure risk includes a history of epilepsy, recent stroke and patients dependent on substances who may seize on withdrawal. In general, more severely unwell patients who require crisis input would not be considered for rTMS.

Side effects

The main rare, adverse events to be aware of are seizures, mania, and hearing loss. Common side effects include mild headache and transient facial muscle twitching during treatment.

Drug interactions

- Use of regular benzodiazepines has been associated with reduced efficacy.
- Sodium valproate has been associated with a higher motor threshold.

Augmentation strategies

- There is RCT evidence that d-cycloserine prescribed for the first 2 weeks of treatment, and taken before rTMS, can be used to augment the effectiveness of rTMS.
- There is evidence that rTMS combination with high-dose levothyroxine (HDT/rTMS) can be effective in rapid-cycling bipolar spectrum disorders.

Further reading

Perera T, George MS, Grammer G, et al. The Clinical TMS Society consensus review and treatment recommendations for TMS therapy for major depressive disorder. Brain Stimul. 2016 May–Jun;9(3):336–346.

Cole EJ, Phillips AL, Bentzley BS, et al. Stanford Neuromodulation Therapy (SNT): A double-blind randomized controlled trial. Am J Psychiatry. 2022 Feb;179(2):132–141.

Cappon D, den Boer T, Jordan C, et al. Transcranial magnetic stimulation (TMS) for geriatric depression. Ageing Res Rev. 2022 Feb;74:101531.

Baeken C, De Raedt R. Neurobiological mechanisms of repetitive transcranial magnetic stimulation on the underlying neurocircuitry in unipolar depression. Dialogues Clin Neurosci. 2011;13(1):139–145.

Zamar AC, Kouimtsidis C, Lulsegged A, et al. A new treatment protocol of combined high-dose levothyroxine and repetitive transcranial magnetic stimulation for the treatment of rapid-cycling bipolar spectrum disorders: A cohort evaluation of 55 patients. J Clin Med. 2022 Sep 30;11(19).

Electroconvulsive therapy

ECT is a proven and generally safe treatment for depression including among older people. The main indication is likely to be severe depressive illness, especially where clinical features include delusions, refusal to eat or drink, and severe retardation, all presentations found more commonly among older people. ECT remains the most effective treatment for patients with this clinical profile. The problems of ECT are no different in older people, but issues to consider include anaesthetic fitness and management of cognitive impairment associated with ECT. Most ECT services have a 'pathway' document which helps the referrer to complete the necessary pre-treatment workup and investigations.

Pre-treatment considerations

- Mental capacity assessment.
- Consent to treatment (incompetent patients, or those refusing but in need of ECT, may require detention under mental health legislation).
- Medications used—particular cautions with benzodiazepines (raise seizure threshold), lithium (confusion and lithium toxicity), clozapine (may lower seizure threshold).
- Anaesthetic fitness, including past medical history.
- Previous anaesthetic/treatment response.
- Prescription of course of ECT by referring team. The initial session is usually for titration.

Investigations

- ECG, U&E, FBC, physical examination, chest X-ray if required.
- Cognitive examination (e.g. of anterograde memory; the MMSE may be too crude for this task).

Day of treatment

- Nil by mouth.
- Reassure patient.
- Oxygenation.
- Record seizure duration.

Recovery

- Monitor during recovery.
- Post-treatment cognitive impairment (reassure) and headache (use simple analgesia, e.g. paracetamol).

Between treatments

- Assess clinical response to each treatment.

If cognitively impaired

- Reduce frequency of treatment.
- Unilateral electrode placement.
- Alternative treatment (antidepressants, psychological treatment).

Rapid-acting antidepressants

Esketamine and ketamine

Ketamine can sometimes induce a remarkably rapid response and provide hope for patients who have not responded to other treatments. Ketamine's multiple, powerful psychoactive effects mean that clinical usage can be complex and has led to it being dubbed in the literature as the 'ketamine tiger'. Ketamine's most well-known pharmacological effect is blockade of N-methyl D-aspartate (NMDA) receptors.

Indications

Esketamine, the S-enantiomer of ketamine, is formulated as a nasal spray and has been granted a marketing authorization in most jurisdictions for use in treatment-resistant depression (TRD), defined as lack of response to at least two other antidepressants (AD), and also for major depressive disorder (MDD) with acute suicidal ideation (SI). Racemic ketamine, the same as used in anaesthesia, is also effective. In general, there is less evidence for esketamine and ketamine in older adult patients.

Patients typically begin with an induction regime, for esketamine this is 56-84 mg twice weekly for a month, then once weekly for another month and then an assessment of response, typically defined as a 50% or greater reduction in a depression rating scale. In elderly patients, the starting dose is 28 mg. For generic ketamine, a variety of induction regimes exist but typically consist of 3-6 parenteral doses starting at 0.5 mg/kg titrated to response. For maintenance, the lowest dose and frequency required to maintain response is prescribed.

Contraindications and cautions

The main contraindications, some relative depending on severity, are aneurysmal vascular disease, artierio-venous malformation (AVM), intracerebral haemorrhage, history of severe cardiac disease or unstable blood pressure, severe liver or kidney disease, pregnancy, breastfeeding, a history of psychosis, urological disease or a history of substance use disorder.

Pharmacokinetics and pharmacodynamics

[38,39]

Ketamine is metabolized primarily by CYP2B6 and CYP3A4 and therefore it is advised to avoid hepatic inducers/inhibitors. Advanced age, renal and hepatic impairment can increase the effective dose. Commonly encountered, and important interactions to be aware of:

- Benzodiazepines may reduce the effectiveness of ketamine
- Psychostimulants (e.g., amphetamines, methylphenidate, modafinil, armodafinil) or monoamine oxidase inhibitors (MAOIs) may increase blood pressure when prescribed with ketamine

Side effects

- Acute: Dissociation, dizziness, sedation, blood pressure increased, hypoesthesia, vomiting, euphoric mood, and vertigo. Patients advised not to drive home after being dosed.
- Chronic: irreversible bladder damage ('ketamine bladder' – unlikely at medical dosing levels), dependence, misuse, hypertension, cognitive impairment (memory, attention, reaction speed and motor skills).

Dextromethorphan-bupropion (Auvelity)

Dextromethorphan is an N-methyl D-aspartate (NMDA) receptor antagonist and sigma-1 agonist. However, dosing dextromethorphan is difficult because it is quickly broken down in the body. Adding bupropion, a noradrenaline and dopamine reuptake inhibitor (NDRI), blocks CYP2D6a and allows therapeutic blood levels to be reached. Dextromethorphan-bupropion combination, like ketamine, has a rapid acting antidepressant effect. Unlike ketamine, it does not produce dissociation. It comes as a regular tablet to be taken at home and is indicated for MDD. The combination of dextromethorphan and bupropion is superior to bupropion alone[40].

Neuroactive steroids (brexanolone and zuranolone)

Another group of medicines shown to have rapid antidepressant action are the neuroactive steroids. This class are positive allosteric modulators (PAM) of GABA receptors. Interestingly, they are the only drugs with regulatory approvals for treating post-partum depression (PPD). The effect in geriatric patients with a diagnosis of MDD is currently unknown. Brexanolone must be given intravenously over a 60-hour period, whereas zuranolone is dosed simply as a tablet.

Further reading

Domino EF, Warner DS. Taming the ketamine tiger. Anesthesiology. 2010;113(3):678–684.

Diamond PR, Farmery AD, Atkinson S, et al. Ketamine infusions for treatment resistant depression: a series of 28 patients treated weekly or twice weekly in an ECT clinic. J Psychopharmacol. 2014 Jun;28(6):536–44.

Tabuteau H, Jones A, Anderson A, et al. Effect of AXS-05 (dextromethorphan-bupropion) in major depressive disorder: A randomized double-blind controlled trial. Am J Psychiatry. 2022 Jul;179(7):490–499.

Managing the recently bereaved

The main point is to know when intervention is necessary. Older people are much more likely to have bereavements than younger people—their siblings/peers are older and those who are currently older people came from larger families.

Normal grieving

Early reactions are disbelief, numbness, shock, and sometimes denial (carrying on as if nothing has happened). This gives way to a combination of anger, sadness, crying, insomnia, appetite loss, preoccupation with the person lost, or guilt (the bereaved person may seek reassurance that they have done everything possible). A significant minority may experience true hallucinations of the lost person. Gradually, these feelings subside as acceptance of the loss occurs, with readjustment of life plans. Grieving usually lasts for 3–12 months—this varies greatly and in some cultures much longer periods are normal.

Pathological grieving

Also known as morbid or abnormal grief, this term is used when grief is either completely absent or is excessively severe or prolonged. Marked hopelessness, strong suicidal ideas, psychomotor retardation, guilt of delusional intensity, or severe weight loss all indicate pathological grief and warrant intervention.

A debate has long existed as to the status of grief—is it a psychiatric disorder or an essential part of human experience? Some feel it is a dismally ignored mental illness, others a necessary part of spiritual renewal. Freud wrote of the similarity between grief and depression in *Mourning and melancholia*. A combination of common sense and experience should make decisions in this area easier.

What to do with a bereaved person

- Sympathize with the loss.
- Understand what is experienced in normal grief.
- Arrange timely review for high-risk people—those with previous depressive disorder, those suddenly bereaved or those socially isolated.
- Look for warning signs of pathological grief—significant weight loss, psychomotor retardation, suicidal and delusional thinking.
- For people with directly bereavement-related distress, counselling at primary care level or with specialist volunteers may be appropriate.
- For those with clear depressive symptoms, initiate antidepressant treatment and/or psychotherapy (first-line supportive type, consider more specialized therapy including CBT if little progress).
- Optimism is appropriate; vigorous treatment of late-life depression following bereavement has been clearly shown to be effective.

Managing depression in frail older people

Frail older people have a number of risk factors for new depressive disorders—physical illness, disability, higher risk of institutionalization. Managing depression in frail older people requires a vigorous treatment approach and awareness of particular problems with treatments. Outcomes of depression among older people with physical illness are no worse than among older people with fewer physical illnesses, despite assertions to the contrary. Very frail older people referred with suspected depression often turn out not to be clinically depressed. Clinical judgement by someone with a lot of experience (e.g. the patient's GP or an old age psychiatrist) is often needed on this point. There can be considerable value in assessing a patient of this type. Value can be added in the following ways:

1. In acknowledging the patient perspective that there is a limited future, and that sadness and even despair in the face of current problems are legitimate
2. Avoiding likely side effects from antidepressants
3. Avoiding unnecessary interventions like nasogastric feeding or intravenous fluids
4. Allowing patient and family to focus on what patient still enjoys and values rather then labelling them as depressed.

Problems with drug treatment in depression

- Compliance issues—reading prescriptions, muddling multiple drugs.
- Swallowing tablets may require assistance or supervision of liquid doses.
- Reduced body mass and deficient renal excretion may lead to greater plasma concentrations and more side effects early.
- Multiple medications may mean higher risks of interactions, e.g. warfarin effect may be increased by SSRIs, which also diminish hepatic metabolism so may enhance concentrations of other psychotropic drugs and antiepileptics, and can lead to CNS excitation when combined with selegiline.
- Inadequate dosing has been a major problem with tricyclic antidepressants—much less so with SSRIs.

Suicide in older people

Epidemiology

Globally, suicide has been estimated to affect 27 people aged 70 or over per 100,000[41]. Methods include overdose, hanging, and shooting. Among older people, completed suicide is more common among men, while attempts are found equally among men and women. Suicide rates overall have fallen in a number of Western countries from 1970s on. This fall has been more pronounced among older people, for reasons that are not understood. The most important risk factors remain male gender, depressive illness, and painful physical illness.

Definite higher risk

- Male gender (3-4 times more likely to commit suicide).
- Depressive illness (at least two-thirds of completed suicides).
- Physical illness, especially if painful.

Probable higher risk

- Socially isolated.
- Widowed (for male widowers; women appear protected from this risk).
- Abnormal personality.
- Alcohol abuse.

No clear association

- Dementia.

Lower risk

- Residential care.
- Currently married.
- Female gender.

Compared with younger people

- Suicide attempts among older people are generally more serious than among younger people. A higher proportion of attempts are genuine attempts to die. When followed up, older people who have attempted suicide (self-harmed) are more likely to kill themselves than younger people. Predictors of completed suicide are male gender, and a history of depression.

Prevention

- Primary prevention—remove lethal means, e.g. banning coproxamol, replacing tricyclic antidepressants with SSRIs, catalytic converters (catalytic converters on exhausts make it harder to commit suicide through carbon monoxide poisoning).
- Secondary prevention—screening for depression in primary care, or among older medical in-patients, combined with education of clinicians.

Managing an older person after an overdose

General principles

- Manage medical consequences of overdose as a priority.
- Assess further risk.
- Identify psychiatric disorder.
- Identify life problems which can be meaningfully addressed.

Background

- In history taking, also get a collateral history from another person (especially family members).
- Does he/she have symptoms of depression (low mood, hopelessness, sleep/appetite/weight disturbance/diurnal variation)?
- Is he/she widowed?
- What are his/her social contacts?
- Any previous history of suicide attempts?
- Is he/she in pain?
- Has he/she suffered recent losses?

The attempt

- Was it planned or spontaneous?
- How long had she/he been feeling like this?
- Did she/he think the method would be fatal?
- Were there any final acts (making a will, writing a note)?
- Did she/he conceal the attempt?
- Was she/he found by accident?

Current attitude

- Does he/she wish he/she had died?
- How does he/she feel about the future?
- How does he/she feel others would be affected?
- Does he/she want to live? Does he/she plan to do it again?
- Are there depressive features in the mental state (agitation, retardation, sad expression, hopelessness, suicidal ideas)?
- Has anything about the situation changed?

Decide risk

- Need to decide if risk is high or low, in the short term and longer term.
- Classic high-risk patient: male sex, widowed, bone cancer, depressive illness, on tricyclic antidepressants, planned attempt, survived by luck, wishes he had died, ambivalent about repetition.
- Classic low-risk patient: female sex, married, spontaneous attempt after stress, mild depressive illness, good support, guilty about worrying family, physically well.
- Do not use risk assessment screening tools to decide management—these are inferior to a proper clinical assessment and may increase risk.

Where to manage the patient?

For high-risk patients, transfer to a psychiatric unit may be needed, in some cases under compulsion. For lower-risk patients, discharge home with support, e.g. family, community mental health team, day hospital, general or family practitioner is appropriate.

Who will manage the patient?

In any case where risk appears substantial, assessment by a specialist (nurse or doctor from mental health service) is appropriate. The specialist can advise on precise risk status and arrange ongoing management. If the patient appears high risk and insists on leaving, compulsion to remain until specialist assessment is appropriate.

Intervene to achieve change

- Treat any depressive or manic illness.
- Increase analgesia and refer to pain clinic if in pain.
- Arrange social support, e.g. day centre, if isolated.
- Psychological treatment, e.g. bereavement counselling.

References

1. Alexopoulos GS. Mechanisms and treatment of late-life depression. Translational Psychiatry. 2019 2019/08/05;9(1):188.
2. Ghaemi SN. On late life depression and mania. Personal communication. 2023.
3. Alexopoulos GS. The depression-executive dysfunction syndrome of late life: A specific target for D3 agonists? Am J Geriatr Psychiatry. 2001 Winter;9(1):22–29.
4. Ghaemi SN, Angst J, Vohringer PA, et al. Clinical research diagnostic criteria for bipolar illness (CRDC-BP): Rationale and validity. Int J Bipolar Disord. 2022 Oct 13;10(1):23.
5. Tomasik J, Harrison SJ, Rustogi N, et al. Metabolomic biomarker signatures for bipolar and unipolar depression. JAMA Psychiatry. 2024;81(1):101–106.
6. Brunkhorst-Kanaan N, Klatt-Schreiner K, Hackel J, et al. Targeted lipidomics reveal derangement of ceramides in major depression and bipolar disorder. Metabolism. 2019 Jun;95:65–76.
7. Mencarelli C, Martinez-Martinez P. Ceramide function in the brain: When a slight tilt is enough. Cell Mol Life Sci. 2013 Jan;70(2):181–203.
8. Beekman A, Boks MP, Dols A, et al. Accelerated brain aging as a biomarker for staging in bipolar disorder: An exploratory study. Psychological Medicine. 2023:1–10.
9. Ghaemi SN. Taking disease seriously in DSM. World Psychiatry. 2013 Oct;12(3):210–212.
10. Minen MT, Dhaem OBD, Diest AKV, et al. Migraine and its psychiatric comorbidities. J Neurol, Neurosurgery & Psychiatry. 2016;87(7):741–749.
11. Parker G, Graham R, Synnott H, et al. Is the DSM-5 duration criterion valid for the definition of hypomania? J Affect Disord. 2014 Mar;156:87–91.
12. Beunders AJM, Klaus F, Kok AAL, et al. Bipolar I and bipolar II subtypes in older age: Results from the Global Aging and Geriatric Experiments in Bipolar Disorder (GAGE-BD) project. Bipolar Disord. 2023 Feb;25(1):43–55.
13. Tavares DF, Suen P, Moreno DH, et al. Distractibility, anxiety, irritability, and agitation symptoms are associated with the severity of depressive and manic symptoms in mixed depression. Braz J Psychiatry. 2022 Sep 19;44(6):576–583.
14. Aizenstein HJ, Baskys A, Boldrini M, et al. Vascular depression consensus report—a critical update. BMC Med. 2016 Nov 3;14(1):161.
15. Depp CA, Jeste DV. Bipolar disorder in older adults: A critical review. Bipolar Disord. 2004 Oct;6(5):343–367.
16. Sajatovic M, Popli A, Semple W. Ten-year use of hospital-based services by geriatric veterans with schizophrenia and bipolar disorder. Psychiatr Serv. 1996 Sep;47(9):961–965.
17. Sajatovic M, Dols A, Rej S, et al. Bipolar symptoms, somatic burden, and functioning in older-age bipolar disorder: Analyses from the Global Aging & Geriatric Experiments in Bipolar Disorder Database project. Bipolar Disord. 2022 Mar;24(2):195–206.
18. Eyler LT, Briggs FBS, Dols A, et al. Symptom Severity Mixity in Older-Age Bipolar Disorder: Analyses From the Global Aging and Geriatric Experiments in Bipolar Disorder Database (GAGE-BD). Am J Geriatr Psychiatry. 2022 2022/10/01/;30(10):1096–1107.
19. Montejo L, Torrent C, Jiménez E, et al. Cognition in older adults with bipolar disorder: An ISBD task force systematic review and meta-analysis based on a comprehensive neuropsychological assessment. Bipolar Disorders. 2022 2022-01-02T00:00:00Z.
20. Moorhead SRJ, Young AH. Evidence for a late onset bipolar-I disorder sub-group from 50 years. J Affect Disord. 2003 2003/02/01/;73(3):271–277.

21. Arnold I, Dehning J, Grunze A, et al. Old age bipolar disorder-epidemiology, aetiology and treatment. Medicina (Kaunas). 2021 Jun 8;57(6).
22. Harrison PJ, Colbourne L, Harrison CH. The neuropathology of bipolar disorder: Systematic review and meta-analysis. Mol Psychiatry. 2020 Aug;25(8):1787–1808.
23. Harrison PJ, Geddes JR, Tunbridge EM. The emerging neurobiology of bipolar disorder. Trends Neurosci. 2018 2018/01/01/;41(1):18-30.
24. Cotovio G, Oliveira-Maia AJ. Functional neuroanatomy of mania. Transl Psychiatry. 2022 Jan 24;12(1):29.
25. Villa LM, Colic L, Kim JA, et al. Aging of the brain in bipolar disorder: Illness- and onset-related effects in cortical thickness and subcortical gray matter volume. J Affect Disord. 2023 Feb 15;323:875–883.
26. Lavin P, Rej S, Olagunju AT, et al. Essential data dimensions for prospective international data collection in older age bipolar disorder (OABD): Recommendations from the GAGE-BD group. Bipolar Disorders. 2023;25(7):554–563.
27. Kavalali ET, Monteggia LM. Targeting homeostatic synaptic plasticity for treatment of mood disorders. Neuron. 2020 Jun 3;106(5):715–726.
28. Mishra HK, Ying NM, Luis A, et al. Circadian rhythms in bipolar disorder patient-derived neurons predict lithium response: preliminary studies. Mol Psychiatry. 2021 Jul;26(7):3383–3394.
29. Turrigiano GG. The self-tuning neuron: synaptic scaling of excitatory synapses. Cell. 2008 Oct 31;135(3):422–435.
30. McKnight RF, Adida M, Budge K, et al. Lithium toxicity profile: A systematic review and meta-analysis. Lancet. 2012 Feb 25;379(9817):721–728.
31. Young RC, Mulsant BH, Sajatovic M, et al. GERI-BD: A randomized double-blind controlled trial of lithium and divalproex in the treatment of mania in older patients with bipolar disorder. Am J Psychiatry. 2017 Nov 1;174(11):1086–1093.
32. Correll CU, Newcomer JW, Silverman B et al. Effects of olanzapine combined with samidorphan on weight gain in schizophrenia: A 24-week phase 3 study. Am J Psychiatry. 2020;177(12):1168–1178.
33. Miklowitz DJ, Efthimiou O, Furukawa TA, et al. Adjunctive psychotherapy for bipolar disorder: A systematic review and component network meta-analysis. JAMA Psychiatry. 2021;78(2):141–150.
34. Krause M, Gutsmiedl K, Bighelli I, et al. Efficacy and tolerability of pharmacological and non-pharmacological interventions in older patients with major depressive disorder: A systematic review, pairwise and network meta-analysis. Eur Neuropsychopharmacol. 2019 Sep;29(9):1003–1022.
35. Bishop MM, Fixen DR, Linnebur SA, et al. Cognitive effects of vortioxetine in older adults: a systematic review. Ther Adv Psychopharmacol. 2021;11:20451253211026796.
36. Smith DJ, Griffiths E, Kelly M, et al. Unrecognised bipolar disorder in primary care patients with depression. Br J Psychiatry. 2011 Jul;199(1):49–56.
37. Lavretsky H, Reinlieb M, St Cyr N, et al. Citalopram, methylphenidate, or their combination in geriatric depression: A randomized, double-blind, placebo-controlled trial. Am J Psychiatry. 2015 Jun;172(6):561–569.
38. Sanacora G, Frye MA, McDonald W, et al. A consensus statement on the use of ketamine in the treatment of mood disorders. JAMA Psychiatry. 2017 Apr 1;74(4):399–405.
39. Heifets BD, Bentzley BS, Williams N, et al. Unraveling the opioid actions of S-ketamine and R-ketamine: Comment on Bonaventura et al. Mol Psychiatry. 2021 Nov;26(11):6104–6106.
40. Tabuteau H, Jones A, Anderson A, et al. Effect of AXS-05 (dextromethorphan-bupropion) in major depressive disorder: A randomized double-blind controlled trial. Am J Psychiatry. 2022 Jul;179(7):490–499.
41. De Leo D. Late-life suicide in an aging world. Nature Aging. 2022 2022/01/01;2(1):7–12.

Chapter 5

Anxiety and behaviour disorders

Anxiety presentations

Anxiety as a word refers to a marked subjective emotional state of apprehension and fear. This can be a normal, even helpful, response to stress/threat. More severe anxiety is a common symptom of a number of psychiatric disorders. When anxiety is the dominant symptom, the disorders are usually classified as anxiety or (sometimes) neurotic disorders. Different patterns of anxiety in terms of clinical picture and precipitants lead to characteristic diagnoses; the pattern within individuals tends to run true over a long period.

Symptoms of anxiety

Emotional

A sense of fearful foreboding, which may focus on a particular object or situation (in phobias) or may be independent of particular precipitants.

Physiological

- Autonomic symptoms include dry mouth, tachycardia, palpitations, sweating, dizziness.
- Muscle tension causes tremor, inability to sit still, headache ('tension' type), muscle aches.
- Hyperventilation.
- Paraesthesia in extremities and feelings of dizziness.

Cognitive

Characteristic thoughts are of negative evaluation ('I will make a fool of myself'), catastrophe, or hypochondriacal type ('I am going to collapse', 'I am having a heart attack').

Behavioural

Characteristic behaviours include *escape* from the situation one feels anxious in or *avoidance* of feared situations.

Epidemiology

New diagnoses of anxiety disorders are comparatively rare among older people. Reasons for this may include a true decrease in incidence, resolution of early life cases, selective mortality, or diagnostic difficulties in patients with physical disease or depressive disorder. Phobia is probably the most common of the anxiety disorders in older populations, affecting 3–6% of older people. Outcomes of anxiety disorders in older people have been little studied; probably fewer than half of cases resolve after 3–20 years. Recent cross-sectional prevalence studies report the following statistics: agoraphobia (4.9%), panic disorder (3.8%), animal phobia (3.5%), general anxiety disorder (3.1%), post-traumatic stress disorder (1.4%), social phobia (1.3%), and obsessive–compulsive disorder (0.8%)[1].

Relationship with other illnesses

The concept of the diagnostic hierarchy is relevant here, given the ubiquitous nature of anxiety symptoms. At the top of the hierarchy is organic illness, followed by psychotic disorders and then mood diagnoses. If one of these conditions can explain the anxiety symptoms, then that should be the diagnosis made rather than using multiple comorbid diagnoses.

Dementia

Anxiety symptoms are found very commonly in people with dementia. These may be found in the early stages of the condition as an understandable reaction to developing deficits or as a direct behavioural symptom of moderate to severe dementia, probably as a result of depletion in monoamine neurotransmission. Up to 80% of people with dementia experience significant anxiety symptoms during the course of the dementia. As anxiety may be a presenting complaint in early dementia, cognitive screening should be carried out in such cases. Anxiety may of course artificially depress cognitive performance.

One possible explanation for the decreased incidence of anxiety disorders in older people is that such cases develop dementia which then 'hides' the anxiety disorder; this theory is as yet unsupported by evidence.

Depression

Anxiety and depressed mood frequently coexist. Anxiety symptoms are very common in depression. Careful history taking to establish which symptoms dominate and which came first will usually decide the diagnosis. New-onset anxiety symptoms in older age should strongly suggest a depressive disorder. Depressive symptoms are common in the main anxiety disorders, especially OCD and PTSD.

The main anxiety, stress, obsessive–compulsive and related disorders

The 'fear based' syndromes involve physiological and neuropsychological response to threat. This includes the phobias and panic disorder. Generalized anxiety disorder (GAD) is a more heterogeneous grouping, originating from various concepts including non-specific feelings of anxiety ('pantophobia') and anxious and neurotic depression. Syndromes following extreme stress or trauma include post-traumatic stress disorder (PTSD) and adjustment disorder. The obsessive–compulsive and related disorders are separated from the anxiety disorders in the latest edition of the DSM due to unique course, genetics, and neurobiological features. Relevant to presentations seen in older patients in this section is hoarding disorder. Impulse control disorders also form their own section in recent classification systems. Of relevance is impulsivity seen in patients taking dopaminergic medications, e.g. for Parkinson's disease. Finally, combining impulsivity and compulsivity are the substance related and addiction disorders. Recently, this has expanded to behavioural addictions, including pathological gambling.

Phobias

Phobias are disorders in which anxiety arises mainly, or only, in particular situations which are not dangerous. The situation provokes a variety of anxiety symptoms and is both dreaded and avoided. Simple phobias are of particular objects or experiences, e.g. dogs, spiders, dentists. These usually arise in childhood and may persist for a lifetime. Social phobia is anxiety provoked by social encounters and is disabling. It usually arises in adolescence. Agoraphobia has a lay meaning of fear of open spaces but refers to a fear of uncontrollable outside situations, often with crowds of people and difficult to get away from. It may arise independently in adult life or after a panic attack; if associated with true panic attacks it is known as agoraphobia with panic disorder. In either case, onset is in adult life, later than other phobias. This pattern is most common in older people, often following a distressing event while out alone, and may cause the patient to be housebound.

Panic disorder

Anxiety occurs in discrete bursts, recurs, and is not linked to particular situations (unless in agoraphobic patients). Attacks are unpredictable, sudden, and very severe. Predominant subsequent fears are of further attacks. Panic disorder was originally distinguished from other anxiety disorders based on its response to imipramine[2].

Generalized anxiety disorder

In GAD, anxiety is chronic and persistent (often described as 'free-floating'). It does not occur in discrete bursts, unlike panic disorder.

Obsessive–compulsive disorder

OCD was previously classified with the other anxiety disorders, but now is regarded as separate. While anxiety may be part of the clinical picture, the dominant symptoms are powerful intrusive thoughts/images which come to the patient's mind despite resistance and a recognition that they are the patient's own, and compulsive rituals, where a sequence of actions, e.g. handwashing, must be carried out repeatedly, again despite recognition that the compulsion is irrational. OCD usually starts in early adult life, and if severe may run a chronic fluctuating course, lasting a lifetime. The key neural regions affected are called the cortico–striato–thalamo–cortical (CSTC) circuits.

New cases in old age appear very rarely, and organic illness or depressive disorder should be suspected in such presentations. A systematic review found that two thirds of patients with late-onset OCD were secondary to organic illness such as neurodegeneration, vascular disease, traumatic brain injury, or infection[3]. A distinction from the purposeless, repetitive behaviours often seen in dementia should be made; such behaviours are found in moderate to severe dementia. Hoarding disorder (HD) is thought to be a OCD spectrum disorder, with two peaks in incidence, one in young adults, and one in the elderly[4]. In the elderly, secondary HD is common (e.g. to dementia) in comparison to primary HD.

Impulse control disorders

Impulse control disorders may present in elderly patients taking dopaminergic drugs, e.g. levodopa or pramipexole in the context of Parkinson's disease. A wide variety of presentations is possible such as excessive spending, reckless driving, binge eating, gambling; in general, suspect any new behaviour which is out of character for the patient and potentially harmful[5]. Management involves reviewing the dosage and regime of any dopaminergic medications. Adjunctive CBT has shown efficacy too[6].

Post-traumatic stress disorder

- Studies of the psychological impact of the great wars of the twentieth century have revealed the characteristic symptoms of this disorder. In PTSD, a significant traumatic event, such as an assault, direct threat, or witnessing catastrophe, is followed by persistent symptoms of
  - ***Intrusion:*** the event comes repeatedly to the patient's mind in the form of images, flashbacks (re-experiencing the original trauma), or dreams.
  - ***Arousal:*** poor concentration, anxiety, irritability.
  - ***Avoidance:*** emotional detachment, numbness, failure to consciously recall the trauma, avoidance of places/situations reminiscent of the event.
- The epidemiology of the condition has been examined. Most people experience a potentially traumatic event during a lifetime but fewer than 1 in 20 have PTSD at any stage. Severe cases often persist for many years and in certain cultures may be suffered without complaint. More severe trauma is associated with higher risk, while direct personal injury/threat increases risk further.
- Among older people new onset is relatively rare. Studies of Second World War veterans show high rates of PTSD. Among servicemen interned in POW camps in the war, 60–80% still report some symptoms of PTSD. Clinical experience suggests that such symptoms may be triggered by lesser but still stressful life events suffered in later life.

Somatoform disorders and somatization

- Somatization refers to the expression of psychological distress through physical symptoms. Patients report unexplained or poorly defined but troublesome physical symptoms which are negatively investigated. Symptoms persist despite reassurance. A distinction is sometimes made between hypochondriasis, where a particular illness is feared (e.g. a person believing that their weight loss and abdominal cramps must indicate cancer), and somatization, in which the focus is on symptoms rather than a feared illness. An underlying psychiatric disorder is often present, usually depressive disorder or an anxiety disorder. When the unexplained symptoms are present in the absence of other psychiatric disorder, a somatoform disorder may be diagnosed.
- Somatization is common at all ages and the prevalence among older community and primary care samples has been found to be 1–8%. Among older people, a very strong association with depressive disorder has been confirmed. Depressed older people may present with any physical symptoms but some are characteristic. These include:
    - Faintness
    - Muscle pain
    - Weakness
    - Heavy limbs
    - Lump in throat

Case example

Mrs Smith is a 76-year-old woman who was widowed 5 months previously. She has been presenting to her GP every week for the last 2 months with fatigue, poor sleep, poor appetite, tension headaches, burning feelings on her skin, and dry eyes. She is convinced that she is going to die of a brain tumour and wants a brain scan.

An approach to management of somatized symptoms in older people

This approach draws on what is known to be effective among younger people with somatization. Older people have a high prevalence of physical illness, so a common-sense approach to management of new or uncharacteristic physical symptoms must be taken. It may be easier for medically qualified staff to tolerate uncertainty with such patients.

Is there a physical illness? Is it being adequately dealt with?

In the majority of cases the patient will be adequately investigated and treated before somatization is considered.

Is there a psychiatric illness?

In depressive disorder, the low mood and biological symptoms such as poor sleep, weight loss, poor appetite, poor concentration, and retardation/agitation usually precede the physical complaints. Patients usually admit to gloomy introspection and are likely to admit to depression rather than reject such suggestions.

Is it being adequately treated?

Antidepressant medication will usually resolve depression, with resolution of somatized symptoms.

Do somatized symptoms need independent treatment?

- Stop investigations and hospital referrals.
- Schedule regular appointments with the patient so they do not need to report symptoms in order to be seen.
- Explain that investigations have shown no condition that they cannot recover from.

Use cognitive behavioural techniques

- Identify dysfunctional beliefs ('headaches usually mean brain tumour', 'muscle aches mean exercise has damaged the muscle fibres') and dysfunctional behaviours ('I will stay in bed all weekend to give my muscles a chance to recover').
- Identify positive thinking and behaviour strategies (e.g. demonstrate that holding a book in outstretched hand causes pain) to show effect of muscle tension: 'Exercise increases blood flow and fitness of muscle fibres'.
- Schedule increasing levels of activity and record symptoms in a symptom diary.

Drug treatments for anxiety disorders

In general, SSRIs are used as first line drug treatment, with benzodiazepines (e.g. lorazepam 0.5 mg when required) helpful for short-term, symptomatic management.

Tricyclic antidepressants

Imipramine was the first treatment shown to be effective for panic disorder. Tricyclics cause significant side effects, especially anticholinergic side effects (dry mouth, urinary retention, constipation), drowsiness, hypotension. In patients with anxiety disorders, very low doses, e.g. 10 mg/day, need to be started with 10 mg increments every few days to tolerable maximum in the range 75–150 mg/day. Anxiolytic effects may take several weeks to be felt. Clomipramine is indicated for OCD.

SSRIs

SSRIs such as fluoxetine, citalopram, and paroxetine have licences in most jurisdictions for treatment of anxiety disorders. Unlike tricyclic agents, the full therapeutic dose (similar to that used for depression) can usually be tolerated early by older patients. Patients need to be warned of a temporary increase in anxiety in first 1–2 weeks. In older patients, particular problems occur with hyponatraemia (severe caution if sodium falls below 125).

Serotonin/noradrenaline drugs

Venlafaxine, an SNRI, is often used in anxiety disorders, including GAD. Among older people a relative caution exists in people with established cardiac disease and blood pressure may be elevated at higher doses (usual effective dose 112.5–225 mg/day).

Benzodiazepines

These drugs are widely prescribed for anxiety disorders despite limited evidence of effectiveness among older people. They can be particularly dangerous in older people, in whom they cause sedation, cognitive impairment, ataxia, falls, and delirium. For this reason, long-acting benzodiazepines such as diazepam are best avoided due to their tendency to accumulate. Shorter-acting benzodiazepines such as lorazepam are less likely to accumulate and cause these toxic effects; their shorter duration of action means they are more likely to lead to dependence. Pregabalin, which has a structure similar to GABA, and binds to voltage gated calcium channels, has evidence for efficacy in GAD[7,8] but has considerable abuse potential.

Buspirone

This 5-HT1A partial agonist is unrelated to other anxiolytics. It has some efficacy for anxiety disorders including GAD and is probably well tolerated by older people. Its onset of action is delayed (at least 2 weeks). It requires 2–3 times daily dosing and its long-term effects in older people (among whom anxiety tends to persist) are unknown.

Propranolol

A β-blocker sometimes used for relief of peripheral autonomic symptoms such as palpitations in low doses, e.g. 10 mg twice a day. The many cautions on its use, e.g. asthma, cardiac failure, may limit use in older people.

Antipsychotics

Adjunctive antipsychotics are used for severe OCD, for example second generation agents such as quetiapine, aripiprazole, risperidone, or olanzapine. For PTSD, adjunctive brexpiprazole has been trialled in combination with sertraline with mixed results so far.

Non-drug treatment for anxiety disorders

- Psychological treatment has a very prominent role in the treatment of the anxiety disorders, more so even than in other psychiatric conditions. The most common treatment techniques are based on cognitive and behavioural theories. They involve the identification of unhelpful automatic thoughts ('my racing heart means I am having a heart attack', 'If I go out something terrible may happen like last year') and behaviours (avoidance of going out, repeated visits to the doctor for reassurance); their replacement with more constructive thoughts and behaviours, and encouraging homework and review. These techniques are usually combined with anxiety management techniques of muscular relaxation and breathing exercises to allow mastery of somatic anxiety symptoms. Variants on these techniques include graded exposure to feared situations in phobia and response prevention in OCD.
- Among older people, these techniques have been subject to few controlled trials. A widespread and misplaced myth that older people are less likely to benefit from such interventions exists. Particular barriers to such techniques in older people may include physical disability, sensory impairment, and cognitive deficits. Cost-effective techniques include group treatment, which suits some older people accustomed to meeting in seniors groups/day centres.

Panic disorder

Anxiety management techniques and psychoeducation are appropriate. Patients may at least require some antidepressant drug treatment to hasten improvement.

GAD

Anxiety management is probably effective but adjunctive drug treatment is often required and there is a mixed prognosis. Example psychotherapies include cognitive behavioural therapy (CBT) and applied relaxation.

Simple phobia

Drug treatment has no role in most cases. Graded exposure to a hierarchy of feared situations with anxiety management and cognitive techniques is the treatment of choice.

OCD

Exposure to the feared situation and response prevention (for patients with compulsive rituals) is the usual treatment. CBT or cognitive therapy are also options.

Agoraphobia

Psychological treatment will involve graded re-exposure to the outside world with anxiety management. Direct involvement of the community team or psychology staff is likely to be needed at home for housebound older people.

PTSD

Psychological treatments include trauma-focused individual CBT or eye movement desensitization and reprocessing (EMDR) [9].

Alcohol in older people

There is a spectrum of use of alcohol at any age, from total abstinence through moderate use and harmful use to dependence syndrome.

Usual quoted safe limits

- No more than two drinks a day for men, or one for women, where 1 drink is less than 2 units (US National Institute on Alcohol Abuse and Alcoholism).
- Under 14 units a week for men and women, spread over at least 3 days (UK government guidelines).
- Some countries have higher limits (e.g. Spain and Italy).

Harm is likely

- Above 35 units a week for women.
- Above 50 units a week for men.
- 1 unit = 1 small glass of wine (100 ml of 11% wine), 1 small measure of spirits (25 ml 40% whisky), or a half pint (284 ml) of normal-strength beer (4%).

Dependence syndrome has no intake limits but the following features

- Strong compulsion to drink alcohol.
- Difficulty controlling alcohol intake.
- Withdrawal symptoms on stopping drinking.
- Tolerance (larger and larger amounts needed to get same effect).
- Neglect of social obligations.
- Persistence of drinking despite clear evidence of harm.
- Reinstatement (immediate relapse into full dependence soon after a long period of abstinence).

Physiological effects of alcohol in older people (versus younger)

- Similar amounts of alcohol lead to higher blood alcohol concentrations.
- Similar alcohol levels have greater intoxicating effects.
- Body mass often smaller so less alcohol can be tolerated.
- Increased prevalence of conditions which may be worsened by alcohol.
- Increased prevalence of polypharmacy so interactions more likely.

Alcohol use and misuse among older people

- Abstinence is more common among older people.
- Harmful use is less common among older people.
- Older people tend to reduce their alcohol intake as they age.
- Cohort effects apply—prevalence of harmful use is increasing with ageing of 'baby boomer' generation.
- Men are twice as likely as women to abuse alcohol.

The prevalence of harmful alcohol use among older people is estimated at 1–3% (Western community samples) and 4–20% (hospital in-patient/out-patient samples). Reasons for the reduced prevalence of alcohol disorders among older people include early death of people abusing alcohol in younger life, cohort effects, misdiagnosis due to masking by other medical problems, and strong social stigma against alcohol misuse by older people.

Alcohol and cognitive impairment

- The relationship between alcohol and cognitive impairment is complex. Alcohol abuse predisposes to important causes of cognitive impairment such as subdural haematoma. Alcoholic dementia is a condition found in heavy persistent drinkers which may be very difficult to distinguish in life from comorbid AD. Significant deficits in orientation, short-term memory, and ability to self-care are all found. CT brain scans will usually show generalized atrophy. Improvement in CT findings, as well as improvement in cognitive performance, have been reported on abstinence. The diagnosis is rarely made and the true prevalence is unclear.
- Wernicke–Korsakoff syndrome is found among heavy alcohol abusers. It is associated with deficient availability of thiamine (vitamin B_1), a vitamin important for the integrity of memory and other cognitive pathways. Characteristic neuropathology in strategic brain areas has been shown, including the mammillary bodies, thalamus, hypothalamus, and periaqueductal grey matter. In the acute Wernicke's presentation, patients present with:
  - Disorientation and general cognitive impairment.
  - Ataxia.
  - Opthalmoplegia.
  - Nystagmus.
- Untreated, progression to chronic amnestic syndrome (also known as Korsakoff's syndrome) is usual and is characterized by:
  - Severe deficit in short-term memory.
  - Disorientation in time.
  - Confabulation.
  - Relative preservation of other cognitive functions.

Can alcohol be good for people as they age?

Much media interest has been spurred by increasing evidence that moderate alcohol intake may have beneficial effects for health. However, many of these may be due to selection bias in epidemiological studies, in particular survivorship bias. Research continues but the following patterns emerge from epidemiological research:

- Alcohol abuse is associated with significant health risks including physical health (liver disease, hypertension, cardiomyopathy) and psychiatric disorders (dementia, suicide).
- A population neuroimaging study from the UK biobank suggests that even 7–14 units of alcohol are associated with brain differences. These studies aggregate MRI images from large datasets to assess for statistically significant structural or functional differences. Alcohol was associated with smaller grey volume matter on MRI[10].
- Additional analyses published in PLoS Medicine suggest that moderate alcohol consumption (over 7 units a week) is associated with higher iron in the basal ganglia which could represent a mechanism leading to cognitive decline[11].

Management of alcohol misuse among older people

Immediate

Physical assessment

Medical complications of alcohol may be found, in particular:

- Liver disease, peptic ulceration.
- CNS: head injury, cerebellar degeneration, eye signs.
- CVS: cardiomyopathy, unstable/labile blood pressure.

Cognitive assessment

Acute confusional states should be excluded. Immediate cognitive assessment should establish the presence of focal deficits and degree of memory impairment and disorientation in time.

Hospital or community detoxification

Community detoxification is increasingly available. Older people with significant concurrent physical illness and/or inadequate community social support are likely to need in-patient detoxification.

Short term

Detoxification

Replacement of alcohol with a long-acting benzodiazepine or [illegible] and [illegible] withdrawal symptoms and [illegible] the risk of seizures. Chlordiazepoxide [illegible] (also available [illegible]) or [illegible] are the usual drugs of choice. Older [illegible] drugs are not [illegible] and antipsychotics should only be [illegible] for [illegible] symptoms persisting beyond the expected period of withdrawal. [illegible] blood levels [illegible] interval [illegible] relapses.

Typical chlordiazepoxide detoxification regime

Day 1: 20–30 mg 3–4 times a day.
Day 2: [illegible] 3–4 times a day.
Day 3: [illegible] mg/day in divided doses.
Day 4: [illegible] mg/day in divided doses.
Day 5: [illegible] mg/day in divided doses.

Parenteral thiamine

Vitamin B (thiamine) [illegible] should be offered to all patients undergoing alcohol detoxification and all patients who have misused alcohol who show signs of:

- Ophthalmoplegia
- Acute confusion
- Memory loss
- [illegible]
- Ataxia
- Hypothermia and hypotension.

Anaphylactic reactions [illegible] are about [illegible] for IM injection about [illegible] million [illegible] the IM route is recommended.

Management of alcohol misuse among older people

Immediate

Physical assessment

Myriad complications of alcohol may be found. In particular:

- GI: liver disease, peptic ulceration.
- CNS: head injury, cerebellar degeneration, eye signs.
- CVS: cardiomyopathy, unstable pulse/blood pressure.

Cognitive assessment

Acute encephalopathy should be excluded. Immediate cognitive assessment should establish the presence of acute deficits and degree of anterograde memory impairment and disorientation in time.

Decide on location of detoxification

Community detoxification is increasingly available. Older people with significant comorbid physical illness and/or inadequate community social support are likely to need in-patient detoxification.

Short term

Initiate detoxification

Replacement of alcohol with a long-acting benzodiazepine or equivalent will reduce unpleasant withdrawal symptoms and reduce the risk of seizures. Diazepam, lorazepam (also available parenterally) or chlordiazepoxide are the usual drugs of choice. Other psychotropic drugs are not appropriate—antidepressants and antipsychotics should only be initiated for psychiatric symptoms persisting beyond the period of withdrawal. Anticonvulsants do not usually reach adequate blood levels until withdrawal has peaked so are inferior to benzodiazepines.

Typical chlordiazepoxide detoxification regime

Day 1	20–30 mg 3–4 times a day.
Day 2	20 mg 3–4 times a day.
Day 3	40–50 mg/day in 3–4 divided doses.
Day 4	30–40 mg/day in 3–4 divided doses.
Day 5	20 mg/day in divided doses.

Parenteral thiamine

Vitamin B_1 (thiamine) is poorly absorbed orally. Parenteral (IV or IM) thiamine should be offered to all patients undergoing alcohol detoxification and all patients who have abused alcohol who show signs of:

- Opthalmoplegia.
- Acute confusion.
- Memory loss.
- Disorientation.
- Ataxia.
- Hypothermia and hypotension.

Anaphylactic reactions are rare; rates for IV infusion are about 1/250 000, for IM injection about 1/4 million. In psychiatric wards, the IM route is recommended.

Long-term maintenance

Alcoholics Anonymous

AA arose in the USA in the 1930s. AA provides a unique support programme based on admission of weakness, wish for abstinence, open self-disclosure, and regular peer support. A 12-step programme model is followed worldwide and groups are very widely available. The model does not suit all personalities but all detoxified people should be encouraged to consider attending.

Specialised services

Community/hospital-based services often accept older people. Practical support and motivational interviewing can be effective in reducing relapse.

Drug treatment

- Acamprosate centrally reduces craving for alcohol and may reduce relapse rates. It has been little evaluated in older people but is probably well tolerated. It needs to be initiated soon after abstinence achieved.
- Disulfiram causes acetaldehyde to accumulate in the presence of alcohol and has been used as an aversive treatment for some alcohol-dependent people. The reaction is exceptionally unpleasant and occasionally dangerous. Disulfiram is contraindicated in people with a history of hypertension, cardiac failure, stroke, or ischaemic heart disease so should be rarely used in older people.

Benzodiazepines

Benzodiazepine use is very common among older people and usually involves prescribed medication. Cross-sectional community surveys internationally show 10–30% of older people are prescribed benzodiazepines. Among older people, insomnia is the commonest indication. Prescription becomes more likely in extreme old age and half of new prescriptions lead to long-term use.

In older people

- Pharmacokinetic changes mean similar doses lead to higher plasma concentrations.
- Pharmacodynamic changes mean similar plasma levels cause greater sedation, cognitive impairment, and ataxia.
- Adverse effects of benzodiazepines are more common among older people. In particular, ataxia, falls, cognitive impairment, sedation, and depression are caused.
- Dependence on benzodiazepines can develop after daily use over more than 6–8 weeks. Shorter-acting drugs such as lorazepam are more likely to lead to dependence. Other risk factors for dependence include use for insomnia (to which tolerance develops), other addictions, and abnormal personality.

Long-acting benzodiazepines

- Diazepam.
- Chlordiazepoxide.
- Clonazepam.
- Nitrazepam.

Short-acting benzodiazepines

- Lorazepam.
- Oxazepam.
- Temazepam.

Proper indications for benzodiazepines in older people

- Insomnia (short term use only: 2–4 weeks, when sleep hygiene and alternative treatments have not worked).
- Anxiety disorders.

Improper indications

- Behaviour problems in dementia (frequently used: there is no evidence that they are effective and they increase risk of falls and worsen cognitive impairment), other than very short-term sedation.

Managing insomnia in older people

Assessment and examination

It is not easy to simply prescribe hypnotics to older people who complain of lack of sleep. Rather, identify the causes of insomnia, including psychiatric illness, ignorance of changing need for sleep, and physical illness; may be directly [illegible].

Education

There are several changes in sleep architecture which accompany ageing. These include reduced total sleep time, more fragmented sleep, earlier bedtimes and waking times (advanced sleep phase), longer time to fall asleep (increased sleep latency), and reduced slow-wave sleep (SWS).[1,2]

Exclude other causes

- Pain
- Depressive illness
- Urinary problems

Sleep hygiene

- Give written and verbal information
- Avoid substances—caffeine, alcohol, nicotine
- Regular sleeping hours
- Environment suitable for sleep (temperature, noise, light)

Non-drug treatment of insomnia

CBT and sleep education groups have evidence for effectiveness, including among older people, but unfortunately these are not widely available.[3]

Drug treatment of insomnia

Drugs should be considered a short-term treatment only. Dependence is likely after only a few weeks of treatment, so prescriptions should not be for longer than 4 weeks. There is some evidence that the [illegible] efficacy, side effects, [illegible] benzodiazepines (for example, temazepam). Drug options include:[4]

- [illegible] positive allosteric modulators (PAMs) [illegible] include zopiclone [illegible]
- Short-acting benzodiazepines include lormetazepam (0.5–1 mg) and temazepam (10–20 mg).
- Melatonin or agonists: there is some evidence that prolonged-release melatonin improves sleep onset and quality in patients over 55 years.
- Orexin antagonists [illegible] the effect of orexin, [illegible] wakefulness. [illegible] benzodiazepines. Examples include daridorexant 50 mg.
- Antidepressants: there is limited evidence of efficacy for mirtazapine, trazodone, and [illegible]; there is some evidence that tricyclic doxepin in very low doses (3 mg a day) is efficacious.

Managing insomnia in older people

Full history and examination

It is too easy to simply prescribe hypnotics for older people who complain of lack of sleep. Readily identifiable causes of insomnia, including psychiatric illness, ignorance of changing need for sleep, and physical illness may all be directly responsible.

Education

There are several changes in sleep architecture which accompany ageing. These include reduced total sleep time, more fragmented sleep, earlier bed-times and waking times (advancing sleep phase), longer time to fall asleep (increased sleep latency) and reduced slow wave sleep (SWS)[12].

Exclude other causes

- Pain.
- Depressive illness.
- Urinary problems.

Sleep hygiene

- Give written and verbal information.
- Avoid stimulants—caffeine, alcohol, nicotine.
- Regular sleeping hours.
- Environment suitable for sleep (temperature/noise/light).

Non-drug treatment of insomnia

CBT and sleep education groups have evidence for effectiveness, including among older people. Such interventions are not widely available, however.

Drug treatment of insomnia

Drugs should be considered after the above steps. Dependence is likely after 6 weeks of treatment, so prescriptions should not be for longer than 4 weeks. There is no evidence that the Z drugs (zolpidem, zaleplon, and zopiclone) are different in efficacy, side effects, or addiction potential from short-acting benzodiazepines (lorazepam, temazepam). Drug options include[13]:

- Gamma-aminobutyric acid (GABA)-positive allosteric modulators (PAMs) (e.g. 'z drugs') are efficacious. Examples include zopiclone 3.75 mg once at night or zolpidem 5 mg once at night.
- Short acting benzodiazepines include lorazepam (0.5–1 mg) and temazepam (10–20 mg).
- Melatoninergic agents: there is some evidence that prolonged release melatonin improves sleep onset latency and quality in patients over 55 years.
- Orexin antagonists: these drugs block the effects of orexins, which support wakefulness. They were developed to allow safe, longer-term use in contrast to the benzodiazepines. Examples include daridorexant 25–50 mg.
- Antidepressants: there is limited evidence for efficacy of trimipramine, trazodone, and paroxetine in insomnia. There is some evidence that the tricyclic doxepin in very low doses (3 mg and 6 mg) is efficacious

- Antipsychotics: dopamine-serotonin antagonists can improve sleep but have a broad psychopharmacological effect.
- Intermittent dosing may reduce the risk of tolerance and dependence
- Do not switch to another hypnotic unless side effects preclude use of the first-line agent.

Further reading

British Association of Psychopharmacology (BAP) insomnia guidelines

Wilson S, Anderson K, Baldwin D, et al. British Association for Psychopharmacology consensus statement on evidence-based treatment of insomnia, parasomnias and circadian rhythm disorders: An update. J Psychopharmacol. 2019 Aug;33(8):923–947.

Squalor/neglect

Any clinician dealing with older patients will come across cases of extreme self-neglect associated with domestic squalor. Various terms have been used to describe such situations. In the 1960s the accurate term 'senile break-down in standards of personal and environmental cleanliness' was used to describe older people in extreme squalor, many of whom had mental illness. The more memorable term 'Diogenes syndrome' was introduced in the 1970s; the term refers to the cynic philosopher Diogenes who reputedly lived in a barrel 2,000 years ago, rejecting possessions. Attention was being drawn in these descriptions to older people with unusual, aloof personalities who lived in appalling conditions but did not have mental illness and were strikingly unaware of their dire circumstances. Subsequent formal investigations of the presentation suggest that half of people in squalor are over 65 years, most have either mental or physical illness, and a majority are in fact aware of their plight. Hoarding disorder (HD), thought to be an OCD spectrum disorder, describes patients who accumulate a large amount of unnecessary possessions such that their everyday function or safety is impaired[4]. It may be secondary to a dementia syndrome and is associated with prior neurodevelopmental diagnoses.

Presentations

- Self-neglect (skin/hair/clothing/nails).
- Hoarding (housing cluttered with accumulated individual items especially newsprint, food containers, personal dislike for allowing objects to be disposed of).
- Dirty accommodation (infestation, excrement, lack of cleaning).

Among people who self neglect

- Older age more common.
- Live alone.
- Socially isolated.
- High prevalence (70%) of mental illness.
- One-quarter have direct physical health problem contributing.
- May have unusual personalities.
- May show unawareness of neglect.

Case example

Mr D is a 72-year-old unmarried retired serviceman. He has lived alone in a council flat for 30 years and has lost contact with his family. He drinks 3 cans of normal-strength beer a day. He rejects offers of social care assistance, stating 'I am perfectly all right'. Neighbours have complained of the smell from his flat and a social worker has observed rotting food, large piles of old newspaper, and evidence that he has soiled himself, has long dirty hair, has lost weight, and wears clothes unchanged for months. Under threat of eviction, he agrees to admission to a psychiatric unit. No mental illness is found, though he has mild deficits in short-term memory and is started on thiamine and advised not to drink. He reluctantly agrees to move into a sheltered housing complex. At all stages, he expresses surprise at the state he had got to.

References

1. Canuto A, Weber K, Baertschi M, et al. Anxiety disorders in old age: Psychiatric comorbidities, quality of life, and prevalence according to age, gender, and country. Am J Geriatr Psychiatry. 2018 Feb;26(2):174–185.
2. Klein DF. Delineation of two drug-responsive anxiety syndromes. Psychopharmacologia. 1964 Jun 8;5:397–408.
3. Uvais NA. Late-onset obsessive–compulsive disorder with religious obsessions. Prim Care Companion CNS Disord. 2023 Mar 30;25(2).
4. Nakao T, Kanba S. Pathophysiology and treatment of hoarding disorder. Psychiatry and Clinical Neurosciences. 2019;73(7):370–375.
5. Zhang JF, Wang XX, Feng Y, et al. Impulse control disorders in Parkinson's Disease: Epidemiology, pathogenesis and therapeutic strategies. Front Psychiatry. 2021;12:635494.
6. Okai D, Askey-Jones S, Samuel M, et al. Trial of CBT for impulse control behaviors affecting Parkinson patients and their caregivers. Neurology. 2013 Feb 26;80(9):792–9.
7. Baldwin DS, den Boer JA, Lyndon G, et al. Efficacy and safety of pregabalin in generalised anxiety disorder: A critical review of the literature. J Psychopharmacol. 2015 Oct;29(10):1047–1060.
8. Generoso MB, Trevizol AP, Kasper S, et al. Pregabalin for generalized anxiety disorder: an updated systematic review and meta-analysis. Int Clin Psychopharmacol. 2017 Jan;32(1):49-55.
9. Baldwin DS, Anderson IM, Nutt DJ, et al. Evidence-based pharmacological treatment of anxiety disorders, post-traumatic stress disorder and obsessive–compulsive disorder: a revision of the 2005 guidelines from the British Association for Psychopharmacology. J Psychopharmacol. 2014 May;28(5):403–439.
10. Topiwala A, Ebmeier KP, Maullin-Sapey T, et al. Alcohol consumption and MRI markers of brain structure and function: Cohort study of 25,378 UK Biobank participants. Neuroimage Clin. 2022;35:103066.
11. Topiwala A, Wang C, Ebmeier KP, et al. Associations between moderate alcohol consumption, brain iron, and cognition in UK Biobank participants: Observational and mendelian randomization analyses. PLoS Med. 2022 Jul;19(7):e1004039.
12. Mander BA, Winer JR, Walker MP. Sleep and Human Aging. Neuron. 2017 Apr 5;94(1):19–36.
13. Wilson S, Anderson K, Baldwin D, et al. British Association for Psychopharmacology consensus statement on evidence-based treatment of insomnia, parasomnias and circadian rhythm disorders: An update. J Psychopharmacol. 2019 Aug;33(8):923–947.

Chapter 6

Paranoid illness and schizophrenia

Clinical presentations—background

Psychotic symptoms include any symptoms in which contact with reality is lost and include delusions and hallucinations. These may be found in a variety of illnesses—including schizophrenia, depression, mania, delirium, and dementia. When particular psychotic symptoms dominate the clinical picture, the terms paranoid illness or (loosely and confusingly) psychotic disorder are often used. The most prominent diagnosis of this type is schizophrenia, while brief psychotic disorder and delusional disorder are also sometimes diagnosed. Among older people, nomenclature is even more confusing. 'Graduate' is a term used for people with schizophrenia who have grown old. 'Late paraphrenia' is a term for a late-onset illness resembling schizophrenia in which delusions and hallucinations dominate the picture, but thought disorder and negative symptoms are less commonly found. Debate continues as to whether these late-onset cases are just schizophrenia with a better outcome, or represent a separate illness.

Recent international consensus on age stratification makes a distinction between early-onset schizophrenia (EOS, age of onset < 40), late-onset schizophrenia (LOS, onset between 40 and 60 years of age) and very-late-onset schizophrenia-like psychosis (VLOSLP) which presents after 60 years of age[1].

Causes of psychotic symptoms among older people

Organic brain disease

- AD (50% of cases have psychotic symptoms at some point in illness).
- DLB (90% of cases have psychotic symptoms).
- Delirium.
- Strategic lesions, e.g. infarction in optic radiations.

Functional mental illness

- Psychotic depression.
- Manic episode.
- Bereavement.

Primary psychotic illnesses

- Early-onset schizophrenia.
- Late-onset or very late-onset psychotic illness.

Medication

- Steroids.
- Dopaminergic agents.

Epidemiology

The lifetime incidence of schizophrenia is about 0.9%. Mortality among people with schizophrenia is increased but may be falling. Including late-onset schizophrenia-like illness, a bimodal incidence may be seen, with peak onsets in early life and among older people (Fig. 6.1). Among women, incidence is clearly highest with increasing age.

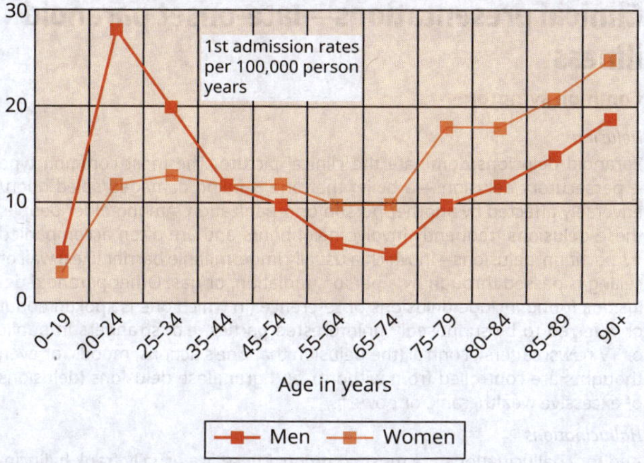

Fig. 6.1 Age and incident presentation of paranoid illness
Reproduced courtesy of Rob Howard, Professor of Old Age Psychiatry, University College London, UK

Outcomes

About half of late-onset cases do not respond to treatment, with 'encapsulation' of delusions (in a quarter) or complete resolution (a quarter) less likely. Encapsulation of delusions means that these ideas remain firmly held and can be confirmed with detailed enquiry. The patient will usually not want to discuss them and will appear able to function reasonably despite holding them. Positive prognostic markers include medication compliance, some social contact, absence of negative features, and a normal pre-morbid personality. Patients diagnosed with late-onset psychotic illness are three times as likely to develop a dementia syndrome[2].

Clinical presentations—late-onset paranoid illness

Common symptoms

Delusions

Paranoid delusions dominate the clinical picture. The most common type is persecutory delusions—a belief that one is being damaged/spied upon/adversely affected by another person or organization. Among older people, these delusions frequently involve neighbours and are often accompanied by 'partition' delusions—in which a usually impermeable barrier like a wall or ceiling is passed through by a person, radiation, or gas. Other paranoid delusions found include delusions of reference (in which one is spoken about or referred to by supposedly uninterested parties, e.g. strangers in public or TV newsreaders), control (the delusion that one's actions, moods, or even thoughts are controlled from without), and grandiose delusions (delusions of excessive wealth, rank, or power).

Hallucinations

Auditory hallucinations are most common. These are usually frank hallucinations and may be of second person (a voice talking to the patient) or third person (voices discussing the patient) type, but are sometimes relatively uncomplicated, e.g. whirring or banging noises or the noise of machines or movement. Olfactory hallucinations may accompany related delusions, e.g. of gas being pumped into one's house. Visual hallucinations are rare and should suggest organic pathology, e.g. DLB or delirium.

Related (occasional) symptoms

Cognitive impairment

In some cases, paranoid symptoms may be the harbinger of early dementia. But for most older people with late-onset schizophrenia, progression to dementia does not follow, and the majority of cases will perform normally on common cognitive tests, e.g. MMSE or MoCA.

Mood symptoms

The relatively benign outcome, and presence of mood symptoms in up to half of cases, have led some to suggest that these cases are in fact psychotic mood disorders. Mild depression, apparently reactive to demoralization about persecution and failure to be believed, is common in late-onset psychotic illness. Careful history will indicate for the majority that mood symptoms did not precede psychotic symptoms.

Uncommon symptoms (never or rarely found)

- Thought disorder.
- Negative symptoms.

Complications

Requests for rehousing, complaints to local authorities and police about supposed persecution, and demands that relatives and friends endorse symptoms, are frequent. Serious complications, such as suicide or violent attack on supposed persecutors, are probably very rare. Neglect, social withdrawal, and suffering due to chronic lack of self-insight are very common and should be considered important risks in planning management.

Aetiology

Personality

Patients with late-onset paranoid illness have long been shown in retrospective case series typically to live alone, be of at least normal IQ, but often to have aloof, paranoid, and schizoid personality traits. Later data from well-controlled studies building pictures of the pre-morbid personality of such cases have confirmed reticence, lack of sociability, shyness, and hostility to be common. Social isolation may follow for such people which makes symptoms harder to eradicate.

Gender

Among late-onset cases, new presentations are much more common among women.

Family history

A positive family history is much less common among relatives of people with late-onset paranoid illness than among younger people. No useful genetic marker has been established.

Sensory deficits

Deafness is associated at all ages with increased risk of paranoid illness and auditory hallucinations in particular. In late-onset paranoid illnesses, deafness has been consistently and specifically shown to be associated. It is presumed that auditory hallucinations become more likely, while relative social isolation through deafness will make delusions become more firmly held, as opportunities to refute the supposed origin of symptoms are fewer, and social encounters are withdrawn from.

Brain changes

Structural neuroimaging

CT and MRI scanning studies have demonstrated in late-onset paranoid illness

- Increased ventricular size can be demonstrated.
- This increased ventricular size is not of a degree useful in diagnosing individual patients.
- Infarction and deep white matter lesion (DWML) are no more common than among controls.

Functional neuroimaging

- Single-photon emission computed tomography (SPET) studies show some hypoperfusion in frontal and temporal areas, suggestive of vascular deficits.
- PET studies have failed to demonstrate primary dopaminergic overactivity.

Neuropsychological findings

- Paranoid symptoms may be found among patients with profound cognitive deficits of dementia.
- No consistent cognitive deficit has been shown in patients with late-onset paranoid illness.
- Prospective work shows an increased risk of dementia.

Management principles

Assessment scales can be helpful in identifying a patient's symptoms and their response to treatment over time. For example, the Brief Psychiatric Rating Scale (BPRS) is a short, clinician-rated questionnaire which evaluates symptoms over 18 questions, rated from 0 to 7.

Assessment

- Establish diagnosis—exclude depression and dementia.
- Identify sensory deficits and social isolation.
- Clarify degree of insight/likelihood of compliance.
- Quantify risk—of neglect/deterioration/violence/suicide/pestering police and social services.

Set goals of treatment

- Resolution of delusions or encapsulation of delusions.
- Containment of complaints/requests for rehousing.
- Building therapeutic alliance.
- Allow ventilation of distress.
- Reduce social isolation.

Compulsion

Use of compulsory powers may be appropriate in the following circumstances:

- Total lack of insight and refusal of treatment.
- Risk of suicide or violent attack on supposed persecutor.
- Risk of serious deterioration if not detained in hospital (and reasonable prospect of improvement on treatment).
- Social threat to patient, e.g. threat of eviction for persistent complaining.
- Failure of all attempts to manage case in community.

Case example

An 83-year-old woman has been widowed for 20 years and lives alone in a rented apartment. She has never had contact with psychiatric services. Her medical history includes only hypertension and an episode of mild hypothermia 2 years ago. She rarely sees her GP and is not taking any regular medication (despite the GP asking her to take antihypertensives). She appears to have no close relatives or friends. A community nurse has seen her at home due to neighbours expressing a concern after not seeing her for some weeks. Her flat is cold and she wears outdoor clothes inside. The flat is in poor condition and she appears to live on tinned food. She is very guarded in answering questions. She is suspicious that neighbours want her 'to be got rid of' and admits that she won't go out as she fears they will get into her flat. She reports hearing noises from upstairs which she feels are hammering or sawing to establish a connection to her flat. The community mental health team visits repeatedly but she will only speak on the doorstep and totally refuses to consider medication or being admitted to a psychiatric hospital. She trusts the community nurse and allows her to take a blood test. This shows anaemia but little else. A decision is made to detain her under the Mental Health Act section 2 for further assessment. During this 4-week admission, she steadfastly refuses medication and asserts her strong wish to be home, though says she would allow community team to visit and assist with shopping. There are very conflicting views in the in-patient team about whether treatment should be enforced. The psychiatrist has to make a decision on this.

Antipsychotic drug treatment

- Antipsychotic drugs are undoubtedly effective in the management of schizophrenia in younger people. A limited number of controlled studies with older people support the use of amisulpiride, haloperidol, quetiapine, risperidone, and olanzapine. Around half of patients will respond to sustained antipsychotic treatment; this modest success rate should be born in mind when considering compulsory treatment.
- Older patients are especially prone to extrapyramidal side effects of antipsychotics; doses should be started low and the atypical class is likely to have fewer such side effects. Reasonable target doses for amisulpiride should be 100 mg daily, for risperidone 2 mg/day, for olanzapine 5 mg/day, and for quetiapine 100 mg/day. Higher doses should be used with caution and with specialist advice.

Non-drug treatment

- Rehousing is a common response to requests by the patient. Evidence of efficacy is lacking; clinical experience and common sense suggest recurrence of symptoms in the new environment is inevitable; such requests should be refused if possible.
- Correcting sensory deficits is a sensible intervention; in particular hearing aids should be sought for deaf patients. Again, evidence of efficacy is lacking but the attempt is at least rational.
- Community team support is likely to be valuable. Allowing visits from a community nurse or social worker may allow opportunities for ventilation of distress, minimize unhelpful complaints to police or housing authorities, and allow monitoring of drug compliance and for deterioration. Social interventions such as day centre attendance are frequently resisted but may allow positive social interactions.
- Specific cognitive intervention is rarely offered—there is limited evidence that insight and social function may be improved in chronic schizophrenia among older people. There is no reason to suppose that CBT used for residual symptoms among younger patients would not work with non-demented older patients, but may be resisted.

Antipsychotic prescribing

Indications

Antipsychotics may be used in older people for the following reasons:

- Treatment of paranoid illness.
- Adjunctive treatment (with antidepressants) of psychotic depression.
- Treatment of mania and maintenance of bipolar affective disorder.
- Management of behaviour problems in people with dementia.
- Empirical treatment for anxiolytic and sedative qualities.

General issues among older people

- First-pass liver metabolism is lower among older people.
- Glomerular and renal tubule excretion are lower.
- Polypharmacy is much more likely.
- Adverse reactions are more common.
- Anticholinergic effects are likely.
- Physical illness is commoner, affecting drug handling and increasing the risk of adverse reactions.
- Older people are more prone to develop tardive dyskinesia with prolonged use of antipsychotics.
- Class effect concern—among people with dementia antipsychotics may worsen prognosis, including by increasing risk of stroke.

Selected drugs

Amisulpride

Amisulpride is an atypical antipsychotic and benzamide derivative. In addition to dopamine blockade at D2 and D3 receptors, it has partial agonistic action at D2 receptors. Whilst it does not act at serotonin 2A or 1A receptors, it does have action at other serotonin 2B and 7 receptors. Typical doses in early-onset schizophrenia are 400 – 800 mg per day. In the antipsychotic treatment of very-late-onset schizophrenia-like psychosis (ATLAS) trial, 101 patients diagnosed with VLOSLP (mean age 80 years old) were randomized to amisulpride 100 mg or placebo[3]. The primary outcome was the change on the BPRS and all participants had a baseline score > 30 points. Amisulpride was chosen because it is relatively non-sedating, and a low dose was selected to minimize side effects. The trial included two stages, each lasting 12 weeks. Patients were randomized to either amisulpride 100 mg in each stage, amisulpride then placebo, or placebo then amisulpride. At 4 weeks, BPRS scores in patients randomized to amisulpride dropped by 9 points and by the end of the trial a net benefit of 8 points compared to placebo was found. Amisulpride was well tolerated. The relative strength of this evidence means that amisulpride should be at least considered for any patient with this presentation.

Haloperidol

A butyrophenone drug in use for many decades. A profound dopamine receptor blocker, it is a highly effective antipsychotic but dopamine blockade in the nigrostriatal pathway makes parkinsonian side effects very likely. It has few anticholinergic effects and can be given orally, intramuscularly, and intravenously. It is still used among older people, particularly with delirium, for this reason. Low doses, e.g. 0.5 mg 2–3 times a day, should be initiated with very cautious increases to usual maximum of 5–10 mg/day. Avoid routine parallel use of anticholinergics to prevent extrapyramidal reactions.

Chlorpromazine

Phenothiazine and the first effective antipsychotic. Strong dopamine blockade; effective but marked antiadrenergic effects (causing postural hypotension) and anticholinergic effects (dry mouth, urinary retention, constipation) make its use among older people troublesome, and it is rarely initiated nowadays.

Thioxanthenes

These drugs—e.g. fluphenazine decanoate, zuclopenthixol decanoate—are often given as depot preparations, e.g. IM injections each 1–4 weeks for maintenance treatment in schizophrenia. This has benefits in ensuring compliance among some older people with chronic schizophrenia. Lower doses than among younger people may be used but tardive dyskinesia is a common eventual side effect.

Olanzapine

An atypical antipsychotic with good efficacy and mixture of dopaminergic, serotonergic, and antihistamine effects. It can be initiated in low doses (e.g. 2.5 mg/day) and increased to maximum among older people of 10 mg/day. It causes a degree of somnolence and likely to cause weight gain. The newer generation antipsychotics such as lurasidone, lumateperone, and cariprazine have lower propensity for metabolic side effects, but most studies of their use have not focussed on older adult populations. There is a lower risk of extrapyramidal side effects than older drugs.

Risperidone

A benzisoxazole drug with significant serotonergic and dopaminergic effects. An effective antipsychotic, it has been shown to have some effect for behavioural problems in dementia and has been a drug of choice for this indication. Recent concern over increased CVA risk mean that it should be avoided for this indication unless a clear benefit/risk analysis has been made. Moderate risk of extrapyramidal side effects mean low doses, i.e. 1–3 mg/day, are preferred in older people.

Quetiapine

Atypical antipsychotic drug with low propensity to cause extrapyramidal side effects. Twice-daily dosing is needed due to short half-life. Doses up to 100–200 mg/day are generally tolerated.

Procholinergic drugs

Several neurotransmitter systems are implicated in the neural circuits which produce the symptoms of psychosis. So far, only drugs targeting dopamine have been efficacious. However, there is now evidence that procholinergic agents might have antipsychotic action. In the EMERGENT-2 trial, a phase 3 RCT, xanomeline-trospium (KarXT), an M1/M4 agonist, was found to be effective in reducing both positive and negative symptoms of schizophrenia[4]. Evidence in real-world settings and over longer periods is needed. For details on pimavanserin, a 5-HT2A antagonist for Parkinson's disease (PD) psychosis, see section on *Parkinson's disease*.

Further reading

EMERGENT-2 trial of M1/M4 agonist KarXT for schizophrenia

Kaul I, Sawchak S, Correll CU, et al. Efficacy and safety of the muscarinic receptor agonist KarXT (xanomeline-trospium) in schizophrenia (EMERGENT-2) in the USA: Results from a randomised, double-blind, placebo-controlled, flexible-dose phase 3 trial. The Lancet. 2024;403(10422):160–170.

Graduates

'Dementia praecox' was a term used by Kraeplin to describe the illness we now call schizophrenia. The term emphasizes the widespread belief that cognitive decline and general deterioration were inevitable in schizophrenia. Remarkably, not until the 1950s was it recognized that older psychiatric hospital populations included both people with dementia and those with disabling but non-progressive illnesses—mood disorders and schizophrenia. 'Graduates' is a term used for people who have had a diagnosis of major mental illness in earlier life and have grown older. Technically the term could apply to any significant mental illness, though usually it is only used to describe ageing patients who had a diagnosis of schizophrenia. Originally it was used to describe people resident in long-stay psychiatric wards, at a time (the early 1980s) when there was widespread concern about their prospects with the impending moves from inpatient to community settings. The outcome was less negative than feared, but this group still all too frequently falls between psychiatric and social service arrangements which do not cater to its needs.

Clinical features

- Patients meet diagnostic criteria for schizophrenia.
- More than one diagnosis may have been recorded in old notes.
- Prominent negative symptoms including social withdrawal, lack of volition, poverty of speech, and blunted affect.
- Inability to self-care successfully in many.
- Positive symptoms such as delusions, hallucinations, and hostility may be found but only intermittently dominate the clinical picture.
- Performance on cognitive tests tends to be poor but progression to dementia is not usual.
- Poor physical health, heavy smoking, and movement disorders, including TD, very common.

Management

- Treatment goals are likely to be limited—complete symptom resolution most unlikely.
- Positive symptoms are more likely than negative symptoms to respond to antipsychotic treatment.
- Compliance issues are likely to be aided by use of depot antipsychotic medication, e.g. flupenthixol decanoate 20–40 mg each 2–4 weeks IM.
- Regular contact with community nurse to monitor compliance is beneficial. Regular assessment of physical health, movement problems (especially TD), and treatment response can be coordinated by community nursing staff.
- Specialist long-stay/rehabilitation residential units are sometimes required for those with severe enduring positive and negative symptoms which mean community living is impractical.

Case example

John is a 72-year-old man who lives in a nursing home. He was first admitted to a psychiatric hospital at age 19 and was given diagnoses of 'psychotic depression' and 'schizoaffective disorder' before a final diagnosis of schizophrenia. His last admission was 8 years ago, since which a community psychiatric nurse has visited him to administer his depot zuclopenthixol decanoate 200 mg every 2 weeks. He had to move into the nursing home 4 years earlier due to self-neglect. He has needed prompting to wash/shave for about 5 years, but he goes into town alone on the bus most days. He smokes heavily but takes treatment for emphysema and angina. When pressed, he admits to hearing voices from the heating system and to believing 'the tax people' are monitoring him, but rarely expresses distress. He is happiest alone, and can only tolerate short interviews. He has an increasing degree of orofacial involuntary movement noticed by his nurse over the last 2 years, but the team and his family agree that reducing or stopping the depot is too risky.

Further reading

Broadway J, Mintzer J. The many faces of psychosis in the elderly. Curr Opin Psychiatr. 2007;20:551–558.

Managing tardive dyskinesia and extrapyramidal symptoms in the elderly

Clinical presentation and assessment

The risk of developing TD is higher in the elderly, especially when dopamine blocking agents have been taken for long durations at higher dose levels. TD refers to persistent, choreoathetoid movements which develop in patients who have been exposed to dopamine antagonists. These can affect the face, the limbs, and the trunk. Sometimes, dyskinesia can present upon withdrawal of dopamine antagonists, which resolves within 4–8 weeks. In this case, the diagnosis is 'neuroleptic withdrawal emergent dyskinesia'. However, true TD continues well beyond this time period. If not adequately recognized and treated, TD can have a devastating impact on patients' quality of life and is associated with significant stigma for those affected. This is important as the use of second-generation dopamine antagonists has broadened, not only for primary psychotic disorders but also for schizoaffective disorders, older age bipolar disorder (OABP), augmentation in late-life depression (LLD), and for the behavioural and psychological symptoms (BPSD) of dementia.

Epidemiology and prevalence: risk of developing TD is highest when using first-generation antipsychotic (FGA) medications, continuous exposure for several years, and in elderly patients. Risk is lower with second-generation antipsychotics (SGA), especially quetiapine and clozapine (or agents with partial dopamine agonist action such as aripiprazole), and with targeted, time-limited usage. One meta-analysis found a prevalence rate of approximately 30% for FGAs and 20% for SGAs, but only 7.2% in SGA use with no prior FGA use[5].

Pathophysiology: Chronic dopamine blockade leads to upregulation (i.e. more) of dopamine receptors, especially in motor striatal pathways. This leads to a dopaminergic super-sensitivity and hence abnormal movements[6]. Therefore, if the dose of the dopamine antagonist is increased, this can block the upregulated receptors with short-term reduction in dyskinetic movements. However, this leads to a vicious cycle of further upregulation.

Assessment

The Abnormal Involuntary Movement Scale (AIMS) is the most widely used, brief assessment tool consisting of 12 items (see next section for the full scale). Each point on the scale represents an important dyskinetic symptom.

Management of TD

A first step is to review the possible causative medication, and consider whether it can be safely stopped or switched to an SGA. The most recent guidelines for TD (e.g. American Psychiatric Association, Maudsley Prescribing Guidelines 2021) recommend a vesicular monoamine transporter (VMAT) inhibitor (valbenazine, deutetrabenazine, tetrabenazine) as first-line treatment because these have licences for management of TD and next-generation agents have been developed. Other options include clonazepam and amantadine. Botulinum toxin has been used for severe, localized, specific dystonia[7] and pallidal deep brain stimulation (DBS) for refractory cases[8].

Vesicular monoamine transporter inhibitors

VMAT inhibitors deplete dopamine available for release into the synapse, thereby reducing dopaminergic neurotransmission. Dopamine is stored in vesicles and enters these vesicles via VMAT. VMAT inhibitors block this process which therefore reduces the amount of dopamine released into the synapse. In TD, because VMAT inhibition reduces dopamine binding post-synaptically to the upregulated receptors, this reduces the subsequent abnormal movements. This also avoids worsening the problem by blocking post-synaptic dopamine receptors with higher doses of dopamine antagonist. Side effects of this class of drug come about if overdosed, and relate to dopamine blockade, for example parkinsonism and gastrointestinal symptoms.

Reserpine

Reserpine, a historically significant drug, is a non-selective VMAT inhibitor, of both VMAT 1 and 2, and due to its effects was used in the treatment of psychosis. It is too unsafe to be used routinely now.

Tetrabenazine

Tetrabenazine is a selective VMAT-2 inhibitor, which has a licence for TD in the UK. Dosing starts at 12.5 mg daily and increases to a maximum of 200 mg. Historically its use has been limited due to its 2–3 times a day dosing and concerns about depression, but in fact a more recent review found little evidence of this association[9]. Next-generation VMAT-2 inhibitors, valbenazine and deutetrabenazine, are based on tetrabenazine's chemical structure and metabolites.

Valbenazine

Valbenazine is a derivative of tetrabenazine combined with valine, and has a licence for use in the USA. In the KINECT-3 study, valbenazine reduced the AIMS score compared to placebo (which resulted in no change) in patients diagnosed with schizophrenia, schizoaffective and mood disorders over a period of 6 weeks[10]. Dosing is 40 or 80 mg once a day.

Deutetrabenazine

Deutetrabenazine is licensed in the USA for TD. Deuteration (i.e. replacing hydrogen with deuterium, a heavy, stable isotope) of tetrabenazine results in improved pharmacokinetics, meaning that it can be dosed less frequently, and a once daily extended release (XR) formulation is available. Deutetrabenazine is titrated up over a few weeks to therapeutic levels[11].

Other extrapyramidal symptoms

If other EPS develop, the medication responsible should be reviewed. For dystonia and parkinsonism, anticholinergics are indicated, e.g. benztropine, procyclidine. Anticholinergics will worsen TD as they promote dopaminergic neurotransmission. For akathisia, in addition to medication review, clonazepam or propranolol can be helpful. Other options include mirtazapine and trazodone.

The Abnormal Involuntary Movement Scale

The AIMS scale (Table 6.1) can be used rapidly (takes minutes) and reliably by clinicians familiar with the patient to rate the degree of movement disorder. Its use avoids the problem of completely subjective accounts of side effects and difficulty in having consistent follow-up by one clinician.

Here is an example AIMS examination procedure (Guy, 1976), see table 6.1 for scoring.

Firstly, observe the patient at rest. Use an examination chair without arms.

1. Ask the patient to remove anything in their mouth, for example, chewing gum.
2. Inquire about their teeth and any dental symptoms.
3. Ask the patient to describe any motor symptoms in their face, hands or feet.
4. Ask the patient to sit down with their hands on their knees, feet on the floor and observe for any involuntary, whole body movements.
5. Ask the patient to sit with their hands hanging down.
6. Observe the tongue at rest, by asking the patient to open their mouth, twice.
7. Ask the patient to protrude the tongue, twice.
8. Instruct the patient to 'tap your thumb with each finger, as quickly as possible', each hand in turn, for 10-15 seconds each.
9. In turn, extend and flex each of the patient's arms.
10. Ask the patient to stand up.
11. Ask the patient to stretch out each arm with palms facing towards the floor.
12. Ask the patient to take a few steps, then turn around and walk back towards the examiner, twice.

Table 6.1. The Abnormal Involuntary Movement Scale (AIMS) Scale

INSTRUCTIONS: **Complete examination procedure (see above) before making rating. Sum of items 1-7 is often used to track change.**	CODE: **0 = None** **1 = Minimal** **2 = Mild** **3 = Moderate** **4 = Severe**	
MOVEMENT RATINGS: Rate highest severity observed. Rate movements that occur upon activation one less than those observed spontaneously. Circle movement as well as code number that applies.		RATER Date
Facial and Oral Movements	1. **Muscles of Facial Expression** e.g. movements of forehead, eyebrows, periorbital area, cheeks including frowning, blinking, smiling, grimacing.	0 1 2 3 4
	2. **Lips and Perioral Area** e.g. puckering, pouting, smacking	0 1 2 3 4
	3. **Jaw** e.g. biting, clenching, chewing, mouth opening, lateral movement.	0 1 2 3 4

Table 6.1. (*Contd.*)

	4. **Tongue** Rate only increases in movement both in and out of mouth. NOT inability to sustain movement. Darting in and out of mouth.	0 1 2 3 4	
Extremity Movements	5. **Upper (arms, wrists. hands. fingers)** Include choreic movements (i.e. rapid, objectively purposeless, irregular, spontaneous) athetoid movements (i.e. slow, irregular, complex, serpentine). DO NOT INCLUDE TREMOR (i.e., repetitive. regular, rhythmic)	0 1 2 3 4	
	6. **Lower (legs, knees, ankles, toes)** e.g. lateral knee movement, foot tapping, heel dropping. foot squirming, inversion and eversion of foot.	0 1 2 3 4	
Trunk Movements	7. **Neck, shoulders, hips** e.g. rocking, twisting, squinting, pelvic gyrations.	0 1 2 3 4	
Global Judgements	8. **Severity of abnormal movements overall**	0 1 2 3 4	
	9. **Incapacitation due to abnormal movements**	0 1 2 3 4	
	10. **Patient's awareness of abnormal movements**. Rate only patient's report No awareness 0 Aware, no distress 1 Aware, mild distress 2 Aware, moderate distress 3 Aware, severe distress 4	0 1 2 3 4	
Dental Status	11. **Current problems with teeth and/or dentures**	No	Yes
	12. **Are dentures usually worn?**	No	Yes
	13. **Edentia (loss of teeth)?**	No	Yes
	14. **Do movements disappear in sleep?**	No	Yes

AIMS Examination Procedure

Firstly, observe the patient at rest. Use an examination chair without arms.

1. Ask the patient whether there is anything in his/her mouth (i.e., gum, candy, etc.) And if there is, remove it.
2. Ask patient about the current condition of his/her teeth. Do teeth bother patient now?
3. Ask the patient whether he/she notices any movements in mouth, face, hands, or feet. If yes, ask to describe and to what extent they currently bother patient or interfere with his/her activities.
4. Have patient sit in chair with hands on knees, legs slightly apart, and feet flat on floor. (Look at entire body for movements while in this position).
5. Ask patient to sit with hands hanging unsupported. If male, between legs; if female and wearing a dress, hanging over knees. (Observe hands or other body areas).
6. Ask patient to open mouth. (Observe tongue at rest within mouth). Do this twice.
7. Ask patient to protrude tongue. (Observe abnormalities of tongue movement). Do this twice.

Continued

Table 6.1. (*Contd.*)

8. Ask patient to tap thumb, with each finger as rapidly as possible for 10 to 15 seconds; first with right hand, then with left hand. (Observe facial and leg movements).
9. Flex and extend patient's left and right arms (one at a time).
10. Ask patient to stand up. (Observe in profile. Observe all body areas again, hips included).
11. Ask patient to extend both arms outstretched in front with palms down. (Observe trunk, legs, and mouth).
12. Have patient walk a few paces, turn, and walk back to chair. (Observe hands and gait). Do this twice.

Reproduced from Guy W. ECDEU Assessment Manual for Psychopharmacology: Revised (DHEW publication number ADM 76-338). Rockville, MD, US Department of Health, Education and Welfare, Public Health Service, Alcohol, Drug Abuse and Mental Health Administration, NIMH Psychopharmacology Research Branch, Division of Extramural Research Programs; 1976: 534–537. Copyright: public domain.

References

1. Howard R, Rabins PV, Seeman MV, et al. Late-onset schizophrenia and very-late-onset schizophrenia-like psychosis: An international consensus. The International Late-Onset Schizophrenia Group. Am J Psychiatry. 2000 Feb;157(2):172–178.
2. Kørner A, Lopez AG, Lauritzen L, et al. Late and very-late first-contact schizophrenia and the risk of dementia—A nationwide register based study. Int J Geriatr Psychiatry. 2009 Jan;24(1):61–67.
3. Howard R, Cort E, Bradley R, et al. Antipsychotic treatment of very late-onset schizophrenia-like psychosis (ATLAS): A randomised, controlled, double-blind trial. Lancet Psychiatry. 2018 Jul;5(7):553–563.
4. Kaul I, Sawchak S, Correll CU, et al. Efficacy and safety of the muscarinic receptor agonist KarXT (xanomeline–trospium) in schizophrenia (EMERGENT-2) in the USA: Results from a randomised, double-blind, placebo-controlled, flexible-dose phase 3 trial. Lancet. 2024;403(10422):160–170.
5. Carbon M, Hsieh CH, Kane JM, et al. Tardive dyskinesia prevalence in the period of second-generation antipsychotic use: A meta-analysis. J Clin Psychiatry. 2017 Mar;78(3):e264–e278.
6. Stahl SM. Comparing pharmacologic mechanism of action for the vesicular monoamine transporter 2 (VMAT2) inhibitors valbenazine and deutetrabenazine in treating tardive dyskinesia: Does one have advantages over the other? CNS Spectrums. 2018;23(4):239–247.
7. Bhidayasiri R, Fahn S, Weiner WJ, et al. Evidence-based guideline: Treatment of tardive syndromes: Report of the Guideline Development Subcommittee of the American Academy of Neurology. Neurology. 2013 Jul 30;81(5):463–469.
8. Pouclet-Courtemanche H, Rouaud T, Thobois S, et al. Long-term efficacy and tolerability of bilateral pallidal stimulation to treat tardive dyskinesia. Neurology. 2016 Feb 16;86(7):651–659.
9. Schultz JL, Killoran A, Nopoulos PC, et al. Evaluating depression and suicidality in tetrabenazine users with Huntington disease. Neurology. 2018 Jul 17;91(3):e202–e207.
10. Hauser RA, Factor SA, Marder SR, et al. KINECT 3: A phase 3 randomized, double-blind, placebo-controlled trial of valbenazine for tardive dyskinesia. Am J Psychiatry. 2017 May 1;174(5):476–484.
11. Anderson KE, Stamler D, Davis MD, et al. Deutetrabenazine for treatment of involuntary movements in patients with tardive dyskinesia (AIM-TD): A double-blind, randomised, placebo-controlled, phase 3 trial. Lancet Psychiatry. 2017 Aug;4(8):595–604.

Chapter 7

Services

Services—overview

Only since the 1950s has it been clearly recognized that abnormal mental states in older people were due to a variety of conditions, with very different outcomes and some eminently amenable to treatment. Since this time, services catering for older people with mental illness have rapidly evolved from asylum-based long-stay ward facilities to a primarily community model of care, parallel to similar developments in services for younger people. A key difference has been the effective withdrawal (in the UK) of the state from provision of long-stay beds for the mentally ill elderly, chiefly those with dementia. Most of this provision now comes from the private sector in the form of care home places. Particularly close working relationships between health and social services are necessary as the need for social care among people with dementia is huge and increasing. The UK is unusual in having comprehensive provision of specialist old age psychiatry services. In other Western countries, management of older people with psychiatric disorders, especially dementia, may fall more to general psychiatrists, neurologists, geriatricians, and primary care physicians, as well as social services.

Specialist psychiatric services in the UK are usually provided by mental health/community care health trusts; most will accept referrals from primary care (e.g. from a GP), from secondary care colleagues (e.g. from other medical specialties), social services, the voluntary sector (e.g. care workers with charity service providers like MIND and the Alzheimer's Society), and even self-referral. UK services have traditionally had some barriers to referral, e.g. the need for community referrals to be made by GPs, but such barriers are reducing. Local arrangements still vary considerably.

Community mental health teams

There are several hundred community mental health teams for older people in the UK, covering almost all of the population. In almost all cases, they cater for older people with the full range of psychiatric disorder, both organic illness, mainly dementia, and functional illness including depressive illness, anxiety disorder, and schizophrenia. Exact configurations differ according to local arrangements but some combination of the following core staff is likely.

Community psychiatric nurses

Community psychiatric nurses (CPNs) are nurses with specialist experience in psychiatric care of older people; roles include screening and assessment in crises, monitoring medication compliance, commissioning packages of social care, counselling carers, and administration of depot medication.

Occupational therapists

Provide expert assessment of the functional abilities of patients and recommendations on how environment (the built environment, care packages, social engagement, assistive technology, activities) may maximize function.

Social workers

May be employed by health or social services. Particularly concentrate on carer support, commissioning and reviewing packages of care, protection of vulnerable people (e.g. financial or physical abuse), and statutory tasks such as Mental Health Act work.

Old age psychiatrists

Medical professionals specializing in the assessment, investigation, and treatment of psychiatric disorders among older people. In the UK, it is likely that around half of new referrals seen have dementia and half have functional disorders such as depressive illness and schizophrenia. The psychiatrist's role is likely to include leadership of in-patient care and more generally of diagnosis and treatment decisions.

Clinical psychologists

Professionals trained in expert assessment of psychological functioning and the use of psychological therapies. Particular roles include neuropsychological assessment in the diagnostic work-up of people with dementia and provision of psychotherapies such as cognitive behavioural therapy (CBT).

Ambulatory care

A combination of concerns about: 1. overstretched hospital systems: 2. reducing unnecessary moves of location; and 3. older people declining in general hospitals after initial treatment, has driven interest in ambulatory care for older people. Ambulatory approaches (often given other names like virtual wards or hospital at home) involve providing hospital quality care in patients own homes. Technological developments have dramatically enhanced the ability of healthcare systems to provide such care. These include remote monitoring, home intravenous fluid delivery, and use of physical observations on home visits, and mean that many hospital admissions can be avoided. The approach has been extensively evaluated, usually with outcomes including functional performance, mortality, or readmission rates. Meta-analysis has shown equal or better outcomes than traditional hospital admission and likely equal cost[1]. These approaches focus on older frail patients but can apply to psychiatric disorders also.

Depression

The concept of home treatment for severe depression is well-established in psychiatric services. For older people with severe depression, reasons for admission to general hospital often include poor oral intake, especially of fluids leading to concern about acute kidney injury, and patients being off legs leading to a need for supervision and assistance with activities of daily living (ADLs) and transfers. Given likely time challenges of recovery from a severe depressive episode (typically 2–6 weeks) in-patient treatment in psychiatric or general hospital may be inevitable. For some patients, even intravenous therapy (usually unavailable in psychiatric hospitals) may be available at home and subcutaneous fluids can also be offered. Psychiatric services always have the option of daily or twice daily visits to ensure medication compliance, orodispersible antidepressants may be available for patients unable to swallow tablets, and home phlebotomy is now widely available, monitoring for biochemical evidence of dehydration.

Delirium

Delirium represents the best opportunity for avoiding hospital care with psychiatric disorder. Many or most significant delirium cases are admitted to general hospitals. This is appropriate for some acute conditions like severe pneumonia, delirium tremens, or epileptic seizures, but for many patients the acute hospital environment is acutely stimulating and likely to make any distress much worse. For care home patients, many of whom have existing dementia, sudden changes in behaviour, sleep, and suspicion of delirium frequently lead to ambulance calls. Point-of-care diagnostics (including blood tests for renal function and inflammatory markers) and domiciliary clinician visits can often mean that a care plan at the care home or even private home can be initiated. Successful admission avoidance schemes may involve provision of extra care assistant staff to help manage disturbed nights in early stages of delirium, to supplement existing stretched staffing. Twelve hours of such time may be equivalent to half the cost of a general hospital in-patient bed. Use of medication to manage distress can be supervised by hospital-based staff. Interventions of this type can only work if experienced clinicians manage cases remotely.

Dementia

Behaviour change when people with dementia are admitted to hospitals is often misinterpreted as delirium. Relocation of such patients to their usual home is almost always a priority. At point of diagnosis of dementia, many patients and families may have an opportunity to state preferences for venue of care in event of future acute illness. Such plans should seek to avoid a pattern of admissions to general hospital, which is associated with a trajectory of faster decline. In cases where hospital admission is clearly necessary, for example fractured neck of femur, most services now emphasize resuming mobility and hospital discharge from earliest opportunity.

Reference

1. Norman G, Bennett P, Vardy E (2023) Virtual wards: A rapid evidence synthesis and implications for the care of older people. Age Ageing. 2023 Jan; 52(1): 2021.

Specialist services—young-onset dementia (YOD)

Dementia is rare among people under the age of 65 years. Among people aged 50–60, incidence (new cases per year) of dementia is below 0.1% compared with 3.0% among those aged 80–84 and 7.0% among those aged over 90. The range of diagnoses found differs significantly. Among YOD cases, AD remains the most common diagnosis, but higher rates of cases of alcohol-related dementia, fronto-temporal dementia, Huntington's disease, dementia complicating Down's syndrome, HIV, and acquired brain injury are found. There may be particular diagnostic difficulty with borderline cases, e.g. MCI, among whom prospective evaluation may be the only option. Particular issues for services providing for younger people include the following:

- **Genetics:** younger-onset cases are more likely to have a strong family pedigree of dementia, whether due to AD, a fronto-temporal dementia, or Huntington's disease. Liaison with, or provision of, genetic counselling is much more likely to be needed.
- **Deficient specialist services:** people with YOD may be inappropriately admitted to day care or residential care with much older people, with whom they have little physically or socially in common.
- **Family dynamics:** unlike older-onset cases, patients with YOD are likely to be working, to have dependent families, and to have spouse carers with severe stress.
- **Physical:** younger-onset cases are less likely to have any physical illness and more likely to be physically powerful. This may present particular risks to the patient and especially to carers.

Specialist services have sprung up to reflect these needs. Many provide specialist day care providing for the needs of younger-onset cases and some provide specialist in-patient assessment and respite. Residential and nursing home care for younger-onset cases is almost always more expensive than that for older people, and specialist involvement in commissioning and monitoring care packages is usual.

Case example

John is a 56-year-old accountant with a wife and two adult children. He presents to a neurologist with a 1-year history of forgetfulness, coarse behaviour causing social embarrassment, e.g. urinating in the garden in daylight, driving while over the limit for alcohol, and making sexually suggestive remarks to colleagues. He has been missing work deadlines and his boss has expressed concerns about accounts he has signed off on as auditor. He is currently suspended from work. He does not admit to any problems and is very reluctant to be seen. He has no medical or psychiatric history. He recalls his father 'retiring early—he may have had dementia'. Physical examination is normal. He allows a cognitive examination by the clinical psychologist linked to the neurology team. His CAMCOG score is 80/104 (usual cut-off for dementia 79) and MMSE 25/30. His deficits are primarily in new learning, visuo-spatial skills, and time orientation. MRI of his brain shows diffuse cerebral atrophy and some particular hippocampal atrophy. Blood investigations are normal.

The neurologist gives him a diagnosis of AD. He is angry when asked to stop driving. The neurologist initiates donepezil and the GP asks for local psychiatric services monitoring. His wife is desperate for some social help. The neurologist refers him to the local YOD team. They see him every 3 months. The consultant in the YOD team writes a medical report which leads to his receiving medical retirement. The community nurse organizes a specialist activity group for YOD sufferers, which John eventually joins. His wife joins a local Alzheimer's Society carers educational and support group and starts campaigning for better services locally. The family are offered genetic counselling but refuse this. On donepezil, he maintains his cognitive performance for 2 years, while behavioural outbursts become less frequent, though he remains irritable with his wife on occasions, eventually necessitating respite he stays at his daughter's home.

Specialist services—old age liaison psychiatry

- Two-thirds of general hospital beds in the UK are occupied by people aged over 65 years. Half of these older people have a psychiatric disorder, most commonly dementia, delirium, and depression. A typical 1,000-bed general hospital would expect to have 6,000 admissions of older people with a significant psychiatric illness per year, but rates of detection and management of these disorders have been low. Psychiatric disorders among older general hospital patients predict poorer outcomes including:
  - Increased mortality
  - Longer hospital stays
  - Increased costs
- Liaison psychiatry services for older people have arisen to meet this need. The liaison model involves a dedicated team, often including nurses, doctors, and social workers, who work closely with general hospital staff to assertively find new cases of psychiatric disorder, jointly manage disorders such as depression and delirium, and plan for future care needs. Education of general hospital staff is a core role.
- Compared with a traditional consultation model, in which individual cases are referred to a general community service, liaison services:
  - Achieve quicker assessment
  - Are proactive rather than passive
  - Have a directly educational role
  - Achieve shorter bed stays

Case example

An 82-year-old woman is described as 'confused' when admitted through A&E to a general medical ward. Her presumed urinary tract infection (UTI) is treated with antibiotics. Ward staff ask for a liaison psychiatry assessment to prepare for move to a care home. The liaison team nurse establishes from the family that she was recently completely independent and deteriorated quickly. Suspecting delirium, she asks the ward nurses to complete twice daily Abbreviated Mental Test (AMT) scoring which shows significant fluctuation. A diagnosis of delirium is made. She is moved to a side room and staff agree to use familiar faces and a consistent style of communication of orientation and treatment information to her. Once her UTI is treated and dehydration corrected, she returns to her normal state and is able to be discharged home with family support only. The liaison team nurse writes a brief report to the patient's GP, advising referral to community old age psychiatry services should mental health problems reappear.

Specialist services—day hospitals

Day hospitals were provided in most old age psychiatry services in the UK but are becoming less common. These allow the admission, assessment, and treatment of older people with both organic and functional psychiatric disorders. A particular focus is on group interventions; groups providing supportive psychotherapy, exercise, CBT for depression, anxiety management, cognitive training, and reminiscence are common. The role of occupational therapy and physiotherapy, both in assessment and provision of activities, is likely to be very prominent.

- The majority of day hospitals provided 10–20 places per day[1].
- Most provide for both organic and functional psychiatric disorders.
- Most patients receive NHS transport.
- Over half of admissions are for over 6 months.
- A third of admissions last over 1 year.

The effectiveness of day hospitals has been questioned. Trials of rehabilitative care in older frail people show no advantage for rehabilitation in day hospitals versus day care or community over day care or home care. No good-quality evidence is available to indicate the effectiveness of psychiatric day hospitals for older people, though patients have been shown to be improved by the end of admissions.

Problems in day hospitals include:

- Prolonged admission.
- Heterogeneity of patient group and reasons for admission.
- Dependency.
- Short therapy hours.
- Insufficient day care places to discharge to.
- Need to provide transport.

Case example

An 83-year-old woman is referred by a community nurse to a psychiatric day hospital for older people. The referral letter states she is 'widowed, lonely and low. She could do with company and structure and an assessment.' She settles in quickly, enjoying company, meals, and group activities. Assessment shows no clear sign of depression and cognitive assessment is normal. At review after 12 weeks she expresses reluctance to try a day centre and her daughter asks that she stay at the day hospital. Repeated attempts to move to a day centre are met with anxiety and weepiness. Eventually a discharge date 3 months in the future is set and day hospital staff accompany her on three occasions to the day centre.

Reference

1. Royal College of Psychiatrists (2001). *Old age psychiatry day hospital survey*. Royal College of Psychiatrists, London.

Specialist services—memory clinics

Memory assessment services (also known as memory clinics) have multiplied in the UK since the 1980s. Spurs to their development included the realization that the vast majority of people with dementia were never known to specialist services, and the need for structured clinics to service the then dawning age of controlled trials of antidementia treatments. Key goals of memory clinics included the early detection of dementia and instigation and monitoring of treatment. Memory clinics vary in emphasis but assessment is likely to include:

- Structured history taking, including from a relative or carer.
- Detailed neuropsychological testing, including instruments such as MoCA or ACE-III.
- Neuroimaging with CT or structural MRI scan.
- Blood test screening for treatable causes of dementia.
- Potential access to newer investigations like lumbar puncture (LP) or positron emission tomography (PET) scanning.
- Feedback of diagnostic information to patients and carers.

It will be clear that these features do not radically differ from more generic services. The emphasis on investigation, early referral, detailed investigation, and exclusion of functional illness leads to different referral patterns. Compared with generic services, patients are younger, have milder cognitive impairment, and are less likely to refuse assessments. Memory clinics appear to lead to greater detection rates for dementia.

Case example

A 74-year-old man, a retired engineer, is referred by his GP to local old age psychiatry services for memory loss. A nurse does a screening home visit but he reacts poorly to this, refusing to perform the MMSE and stating 'there is no point to this, you are making me feel like a child'. The nurse refers him to a memory clinic at a local general hospital, jointly run by the geriatricians and old age psychiatrists. He is willing to come to clinic. He is interviewed by a trainee doctor, has an MoCA done by a psychologist and a full dementia blood screen. An MRI brain scan is booked for 2 weeks later and he returns to memory clinic to receive results after a month. The results are fed back to his wife and him; these indicate early AD. He reluctantly accepts this information but agrees to participate in a local research project which follows people with AD prospectively. He agrees to try an acetylcholinesterase inhibitor (AChEI) and to return to memory clinic in 4 months.

Care homes

One of the responses to a steadily ageing population in Western countries in the latter part of the twentieth century was the expansion in the number of care home places for older people. This was partly driven by the closure of long-stay state care homes and hospital beds and partly by commercial entrepreneurism. In the UK, around 450,000 places are available in care homes for older people. This represents about 5% of all older people. The care home population may have peaked in the last decade, possibly due to policies to deliver care in recipients' own homes where possible.

Mental disorders in care homes

- The majority of people living in care homes have some form of psychiatric disorder. Repeated surveys show that over half of all care home residents have dementia, including in care homes specializing in the care of physical frailty. This figure approaches 100% in care homes specializing in dementia care.
- The prevalence of clinically significant depression, among non-demented residents, has been shown to be 20–40%. Incidence of depression (new cases) is about 5–10% per year. Treatment of depression among care home residents is inadequate and outcomes are often very poor, fewer than half of new cases resolving within a year. Specialist services often do not liaise with care homes unless specific referrals are made, but the ability to detect and understand psychiatric disorder is low among care home staff.
- Older people entering care homes come from acute hospital beds in a half of cases. Decisions are often made quickly and with minimal choice for the older person and their carers. Decisions are often irreversible; under half of those admitted to care homes are likely ever to leave institutional care.
- People with dementia live longer in care homes than non-demented new entrants, reflecting their better physical health. Particular concern has been raised about over-medication in care homes. Surveys in Europe and the USA in the 1980s and 1990s showed multiple psychotropic prescriptions, use of high-dose major tranquilizers, and oversedation to be common. Legislation, national warnings over specific drug side effects, and pharmacy involvement have all been shown to reduce inappropriate use of psychotropic medication in care homes.
- In some countries, especially the Netherlands, specialist medical services for care home residents have been established.

Case example

A 78-year-old woman loses her husband. Her daughters have had to take over a lot of care, including paying bills, cooking, and laundry. Her husband had probably covered up her cognitive impairment for some time. She falls and fractures her neck of femur. After successful surgery, she rehabilitates fairly well on a surgical ward. Her family express concern they can't cope at home and social services indicate that they cannot provide sufficient care to keep her safe. Under pressure from the bed manager, the hospital social worker finds two care home places, one out of her home town and away from family. The family visit on a Thursday evening and feel compelled to accept the other place. She is admitted there the following day. She settles reasonably but continually asks 'when am I going home?' She survives 18 months, declining in the final 6 months with poor appetite, weight loss, going off her legs, and 'giving up' in the words of the carers. No referral to psychiatric services is made.

Services to care homes

Some local services in the UK provide specialist liaison to care homes. This may include reviewing all cases in a care home, training of care home staff, screening for dementia and depression, intensive involvement in management of behaviour disturbance in individual residents, or even taking over the clinical leadership of failing care homes. More commonly, a care home will engage a GP to provide general medical services. Involvement of mental health services will then depend on referral of such cases by GPs.

Netherlands model of care

In the Netherlands, around 57,000 nursing home places are offered. These units are typically large, averaging 200 places each. Since 1989, a new medical specialty of nursing home physicians has been introduced. Around 1,000 such physicians have since had a specialist 2-year training in physical medicine, psychogeriatric assessment, and limitation of handicap. The role is probably unique. Direct costs of the service are probably offset by reduced costs from hospitalization.

Further reading

Royal College of Psychiatrists (2005). *Who cares wins*. London, Royal College of Psychiatrists.

Chapter 8

Ethical and legal issues

Legislation developments

The frequency of mental disorder among older people, and the much higher frequency of vulnerability—to neglect, fraud, deterioration, and isolation, means that in all countries, legislation is commonly considered as a way of compelling care. Whatever legislation is used, central to its use will be the concept that a mental disorder has robbed someone of the ability to make good choices about their care (e.g. whether to accept treatment, or where to live, or whether to accept a care package). In England and Wales, the Mental Health Act and the Deprivation of Liberty Safeguards (DoLs) of the Mental Capacity Act (MCA) are commonly used.

Deprivation of Liberty safeguards

DoLs are part of the MCA (2005). A standard authorization is to a local authority and lasts 12 months. Often, an urgent authorization is needed and lasts 7 days, authorized by the supervising body, e.g. a hospital. DoLs are very commonly used in hospitals and care homes, especially with people with dementia or delirium. DoLs allow supervisors (e.g. hospital nurses or care home managers) to prevent an older person from leaving and to use restraint if needed. The principles are that a person is incapacitated, is subject to continuous supervision of control, and is not free to leave permanently. The tests for using DoLs are

1. The person is over 18 years old.
2. The person has a mental disorder.
3. Mental capacity has been assessed as absent.
4. A best interests assessment has taken place and the deprivation of liberty has been found to be in their interests.
5. The person is eligible, i.e. not already detained under the Mental Health Act.
6. There is no refusal already, e.g. via an advance decision, lasting power of attorney, or deputy appointed by the court of protection.

Liberty Protection Safeguards

Liberty protection safeguards (LPS) have been proposed for England and Wales and will replace DoLs. They have been introduced as DoLs procedures are bureaucratic and involve long delays. LPS were passed into law in 2019, but their introduction has been delayed significantly by COVID and later legislative delays. LPS principles are the same as those for DoLs. Unlike DoLs, they will apply to anyone over 16 years old, will not only apply to hospitals and care homes but also to shared and supported accommodation and also private accommodation. LPS will need to be authorized by 'the responsible body' which now includes health authorities (not just local authorities). Authorizations will last 1 year and may be renewed.

The Mental Health Act

The Mental Health Act 1983 applies to England and Wales (see below for relevant sections). A new draft bill was published in 2022 and proposes:

- To refine mental disorder so that autistic spectrum disorder and learning disability patients cannot be detained under section 3.
- To increase the threshold for detention.

- That nearest relative will be replaced by a nominated person decided by the patient.
- There will be increased access to advocacy.
- Prisons/cells could no longer be considered places of safety.
- A new supervised discharge will be introduced, and a legal maximum of 28-days wait till transfer to hospital from prison.

Many of these changes will lead to little change in practice for older patients with psychiatric disorder. Further changes to the bill may be important for older people, especially if a proposal to introduce statutory advanced choice documents is confirmed.

Capacity/competence—general principles

- Capacity is a legal concept technically meaning the ability to enter into a contract. It has the same meaning as the clinical concept of competence. Healthcare professionals, especially doctors, are frequently called upon to make judgements about capacity. Particular expertise is expected from those who specialize in dementia care, e.g. old age psychiatrists, In many countries, including the UK, an assumption is made that adults have capacity. It is also widely recognized that certain groups in society are likely to lack capacity to make important decisions; these may include children, those with learning disability, and, among older people, those with dementia. Among adults, older people are much more likely to lack capacity, mainly due to the much higher prevalence of dementia in old age. Particular legislation is available in some countries to assist in making decisions about capacity (e.g. the MCA 2005 in England and Wales), while professional bodies offer advice and guidance to members and the public (e.g. the General Medical Council in the UK).
- A number of important decisions likely to be made in late life lead to queries about capacity. These include capacity to make a will, capacity to consent to a medical procedure, capacity to manage financial affairs, capacity to appoint someone as an agent (e.g. donating lasting power of attorney), capacity to decide to remain at home rather than move to a care home. For people lacking capacity, various clinical and legislative options are available. A general principle is that staff will always act in the best interests of the patient.

MCA (2005) test of capacity

- Does the person have an impairment of, or a disturbance in the functioning of, their mind or brain?
- Does the impairment or disturbance mean that the person is unable to make a specific decision when they need to?

General fundamentals of capacity to make a decision

A person with capacity should:

- Understand the decision to be made.
- Believe information given.[1]
- Understand the alternative choices and their consequences.
- Retain information long enough to decide.
- Weigh up the options.
- Communicate a decision.
- Not be subject to undue influence.[1]

1 Part of traditional assessment of capacity; not strictly necessary for current (England and Wales) definition of capacity within the MCA 2005.

Tips for those assessing capacity

Capacity should be assumed

It is not acceptable to assume a lack of capacity in an individual. UK law is quite clear: adults are assumed to have capacity until proven otherwise. Any professional making a judgement about capacity has to give the reasons why they believe capacity is not present. It is unfortunately common for an assumption to be made that people with dementia lack capacity to make important decisions. In reality, in early dementia, capacity is retained or may be regained with reasonable effort by the assessor.

Capacity for one decision does not imply capacity for another

It is sometimes mistakenly believed that a person either has or does not have capacity to make important decisions, i.e. they are either competent or incompetent. In fact, an individual may have capacity to make one decision (e.g. to accept a particular drug or operation) but simultaneously lack capacity for another decision (e.g. to make a will). Capacity must be judged for each decision to be made. There are of course people (e.g. those with advanced dementia) who lack all capacities; the assessor should still state the reasons why capacities are absent.

Capacity can change in an individual

Capacity can vary considerably in a short space of time. Rehydrating an elderly person admitted from home with self-neglect, treating a chest infection which has caused delirium, going back to see a newly admitted patient after a period of rest, or simply waiting a few days or weeks before seeing a borderline case again may lead to a different assessment of capacity.

Do everything possible to increase capacity

The assessor should make sure that medical problems interfering with capacity are resolved, e.g. dehydration/infection/pain. Excessive sedation should be reduced. Severe depression should be treated before decisions are made about capacity. Full information about the decision should be given in a manner understandable to the patient. If at all possible, discussions should take place in a quiet room with minimal distraction.

Maximize information

The professional assessing capacity needs to ensure they know the relevant facts. What are the financial circumstances of the patient? What is the family structure? What are the actual risks inherent in going home from hospital rather than to a care home? What were the wishes of the person expressed throughout their life? What are the wishes of the nearest relatives?

Establish the expressed wishes of the patient

Find out what the patient would have wanted. Have they written an advanced directive? Have they repeatedly expressed a particular wish when well? These matters will assist in deciding on best interests rather than on capacity *per se*.

Does anything influence capacity?

If the person has a mental illness, might it affect capacity? For people with dementia, is the memory deficit and deterioration in judgement and concentration sufficient to mean they cannot understand, retain, or weigh up the information given? For people with paranoid delusions, do the delusions influence their choice of where to live or to whom to leave assets in a will? Mentally ill people may well retain capacity for the decision at hand.

Is there undue external influence?

Might a person or persons be influencing a vulnerable person unduly? Could they have forced them to sign a will? Could they clearly benefit from a particular decision? In many cases an interested party (e.g. a child) would of course benefit from a decision but there will be no evidence of undue influence.

Capacity to make a will

This capacity is known as testamentary capacity. Doctors may be asked to witness a will. It is probably wise to avoid this unless the doctor is confident that the person signing the will has capacity and the doctor is willing to say so in a court of law. The most common scenario where this capacity may be questioned arises when an older person has made a will which excludes someone who may reasonably have expected to benefit. This person may challenge the will on the grounds that the person with dementia lacks testamentary capacity. It is much easier to argue on these matters if the capacity is clearly established prospectively; that is, by an examination of the patient at or around the time of making the will. Deciding on capacity retrospectively on the basis of contemporaneous notes is likely to be very difficult and contentious. Old age psychiatrists are quite frequently asked to comment on this capacity for people with dementia in the UK. The criteria for testamentary capacity have been clearly established in English law since 1870. They are:

The patient should understand the nature of the act

The patient needs to know they are signing a will and that this will decide what happens to their assets after their death. They also need to understand that the new will replaces any old one so should understand how the new will differs.

The patient should understand the extent of their estate

They need to know what they have to leave. This doesn't mean knowing the exact values of a bank account, investment, or house, but the patient needs to be aware of what their main assets are, including a house and any major investments.

The patient needs to know who has claims upon their estate

Specifically, who is being included and excluded. For example, the patient should be able to identify any first-degree relative such as a spouse or children. They should be able to state why individuals are being disinherited. It does not matter if the decision appears foolish or capricious, only that they are aware who might benefit and give a non-delusional reason for exclusion.

Case example

A 82-year-old man has a mild case of dementia, diagnosed 18 months previously. He is widowed and has four children. One was long estranged but has come back to live with his father after 30 years. The father rewrites his will to exclude the other three children, who object. It is clear to the family solicitor that there is a major rift between the children. The solicitor writes to the old age psychiatrist who monitors the patient's care. The instructions given include a request to judge capacity to make a will and a statement of the criteria for these. The solicitor also informs her that the man owns a house worth about £400,000, about £25,000 in shares, and about £14,000 in savings. The old age psychiatrist last saw the patient 4 months previously. MMSE at that time was 19. There was no evidence of delusions but the patient was being cared for by the original three children. She can't make a full judgement just from the notes so arranges to visit him again. At interview, he states clearly that he knows what a will is and says his assets are 'my house... I reckon it's worth £300,000' and 'some shares and about £10,000 in the bank'. He states he knows the other three are fed up but his son who returned 'is like a prodigal... the others are well set in life; they don't need the money'. 'They will come round eventually, I hope.' She writes to the solicitor to conclude that he does have testamentary capacity. This case illustrates the value of careful contemporaneous notes in deciding on capacity.

Capacity to make health care decisions

Two-thirds of people in general hospital beds in the UK are over 65 years old, a pattern found in most developed countries. Older people are much more likely to need invasive and/or serious procedures, so capacity to decide whether to have a procedure is commonly assessed. Doubt about this capacity is particularly likely when very frail or demented older people require serious procedures, e.g. percutaneous endoscopic gastrostomy (PEG) tube insertion, ECT, or major surgery. For common procedures such as accepting medication, having a blood test, or being physically examined, simple verbal consent, whether explicit or tacit (consent assumed as no objection is made) is acceptable. For the more significant procedures, explicit criteria should be met, as outlined below. A common error is to assume that a signed consent form means informed consent was obtained; it in fact records no more than a discussion having occurred.

To give informed consent the patient should:

Understand why a procedure is proposed

They need to understand what condition the procedure is for. It is not necessary that they be exact about this, e.g. a patient saying 'bad infection' when they have *Clostridium difficile* sepsis may be sufficient in many cases.

Understand the nature of the procedure

They need to know what procedure will be done. For example, ECT needs to be understood as electrical treatment under anaesthetic which works by causing a short seizure.

Understand the choice available

They need to know what the alternatives to the treatment are, including no treatment. Understanding that they have a choice of surgery, or chemotherapy for cancer, with no treatment being their ultimate choice, usually suffices.

Understand the benefits and risks of each course of action

They need to be aware in broad terms of the consequences of each choice. It isn't necessary for them to know 5-year survival rates in breast cancer surgical options, but knowing that a radical mastectomy may carry a longer survival than local surgery is needed.

Believe the information given

Patients with severe depression may believe that they are doomed whatever the choice made, or patients with schizophrenia may believe themselves conspired against. Every effort should be made to establish whether mental illness may directly affect the cognitive processes necessary to give informed consent. This may not affect the legal test of capacity of the 2005 MCA, but is an important principle in medical consent.

Retain the information for long enough to make a decision

Patients with dementia may be unable to explain the main points back after, say, 5 min; retention of details for hours or days is not needed but the minutes for weighing up and deciding are important. It is wise to retest (if necessary giving the information again) in doubtful cases.

Weigh it up and communicate a decision

The patient should be able to judge pros and cons and be able to indicate clearly what choice they have made, by whatever means.

Case example

A man aged 84 years with established dementia is admitted to a geriatric ward with falls and poor eating. He refuses all food and fluids and won't take medication. An old age psychiatrist is asked to 'authorize' a PEG tube. The patient has persistently stated that he wants to die to join his wife. He has refused most food and care from home carers for a year. When asked what will happen if he carries on he says 'I will die'. He is not clinically depressed. He knows that the procedure is 'a tube in my stomach to give me stuff'. His MMSE is 18 on the ward. The old age psychiatrist sees him again the next day but his views are unchanged. The psychiatrist writes in the medical notes that 'this man has undoubted dementia but understands the procedure, the reasons for it and what will happen if he carries on without it. He is adamant he does not want it and is not in my view clinically depressed. I believe he has capacity to decide on this issue and that therefore a PEG tube cannot be inserted.'

Capacity to make social care decisions

Many older people may be fiercely independent, even in the face of mounting evidence that they will need more social care. In hospital, the most common dilemma involves an older person, usually with dementia, who faces obvious risks if they go home but insists they do not want to enter a care home. In the community, the same situation applies, in which older people refuse either care being introduced to them at home or to enter a care home. These situations involve risk, and doctors may be asked to comment on the person's capacity to decide this. One common misconception is that any risk is unacceptable. There is in fact no risk-free circumstance, just greater and lesser risk. Deciding that someone lacks capacity does not automatically mean that compulsion is justified; a careful weighing of the risks of not introducing care versus the distress of forcible care, e.g. in a care home, should be made for each individual.

Patients should:

Understand what care is proposed

For example, that a move to a care home is needed, or that a carer will come in twice a day to ensure medication is taken and that they have a hot meal.

Understand why care is needed

This equates to some appreciation of risk—the older person may flatly deny an obvious risk, while another may acknowledge that they may fall but they still don't want to leave home.

Understand the consequences of decision

Appreciate what will happen if they accept the care and if they refuse it. For example, in a care home they may fall just as often as at home but at least someone will be around to pick them up. Accepting a home carer may mean they will take their tablets regularly, and they may need them to control pain.

Professionals should ponder:

Has every alternative been explored?

The least restrictive option should be explored. Negotiation will often lead to voluntary admission to a care home or acceptance of partial care, e.g. a carer visiting once a day may allow them to trust more frequent visitors.

What will cause the most distress?

A weighing of relative risk and distress to patient/family/professional carers (if they stay at home) versus distress to the patient (if they are compelled into care) should be made.

Case example

A 90-year-old lady is frail and may have cognitive impairment; she has never been diagnosed with dementia. She lives alone and wants 'to die at home'. The carers organized by her social worker find blood on her sheets every day (she has a probable rectal carcinoma but is not considered a candidate for active treatment) and she is losing weight, eating very little. The social worker calls her GP out to see her, asking that she be forcibly admitted to a care home. The GP has known her a long time. She is a committed Christian and says 'I look forward to dying'. She scores 23/30 on MMSE. She says 'I know I can't look after myself but I want to end my days at home'. The social worker is unwilling to take further risks and the GP reluctantly calls for an MHA assessment. The lady is removed to a care home under guardianship arrangements and dies, unhappy, 11 days later.

Financial capacity

Much concern is often expressed about the ability of older people to manage their financial affairs. These abilities are focused on in old age for a number of reasons; these include sensory deficits, frailty due to physical illness, increased prevalence of dementia, and the reality of major financial decisions such as paying for care or making a will. There is no standard established method for testing financial capacity. Indeed, one cannot speak of a general capacity for financial decision-making; rather an individual may or may not have capacity for an individual decision. The capacity to manage the transaction of buying a newspaper is clearly not the same as that required to negotiate the sale of a house.

The questions below cover a range of abilities relevant to financial decision-making in old age; it will be clear that financial capacity is not 'all or nothing' and capacity in these areas will vary among both cognitively impaired and cognitively intact older people.

- Does the person have basic skills to manage money—identifying currency, adding notes/coins by value?
- Can the person correctly state what change they would expect for one or more items of differing value?
- Can they understand what a bank account, a cheque book, a cash card, and a credit card are?
- Can they tell you what a direct debit and a standing order are?
- Can they explain the parts of their bank statement?
- Can they identify solicitation by advert (post/email) for legitimate and bogus (spam) financial transactions?

In dealing with lack of financial capacity, use of legal manoeuvres may be unnecessary. Family members often take over financial affairs such as paying bills, which are now commonly paid by direct debit, reducing the number of transactions needed. Family will often also supervise shopping. In disputed cases, many jurisdictions allow for an agent to be appointed to manage financial affairs. Common sense holds that this should be done in advance of incapacity supervening. In England and Wales, a power known as lasting power of attorney (LPA) could be signed over, usually to a close relative, which is signed by a person in full capacity and registered after capacity is lost, e.g. after stroke or dementia develops. In practice, even those who have signed powers of attorney in England and Wales are often not registered even after the individual becomes incapacitated.

Conditions for donating LPA

The donor (the patient) must understand that:

- The attorney will be able to assume complete control over the donor's affairs.
- The attorney will be able to do almost anything with the donor's money which the donor would have done in the past.

- The attorney's power will continue after the donor becomes incapable, by reason of mental disorder, of managing their money and property.
- The donor can in such circumstances never reverse the power.

It will be clear that some people with dementia do not have this capacity; the test of capacity is a stringent one as the stakes are high. But it remains the case that many people with dementia do have this capacity, even if they lack capacity to make financial decisions.

The Mental Capacity Act (2005)

In the UK, a combination of case law and specific courts have governed dealings with incapacitated persons. The situation left very wide scope for doctors to act in the 'best interests' of patients. Courts dealt primarily with financial competence issues and emergency cases. In Scotland, the Adults with Incapacity (Scotland) Act 2000 is in force, and in 2007 the MCA (2005)[1] came into legal force for England and Wales. The latter act expands existing court powers to include healthcare as well as financial decision-making, clarifies exactly who can make what decisions and when, and introduces mandatory procedures for assessing capacity. Five principles underlie the act:

- A presumption of capacity.
- The right for individuals to be supported in making decisions.
- Individuals retain the right to make unusual decisions, however unwise.
- Best interests will always determine what is done for incapacitated persons.
- The least restrictive option is always sought for those without capacity.

Assessing capacity

A single test is done for capacity to make one decision at one time; there will be no presumption of incapacity based on age, appearance, or diagnosis.

Best interests

The Act provides a checklist for deciding what is in an individual's best interests. Those assessing it must consider any advance directive/written statement made by the person and must consult with carers or family members.

Acts in connection with care/treatment

The Act clarifies that no clinician/carer would be legally liable for actions like injection or restraint (technically, a deprivation of liberty) if they had carefully considered capacity and best interests and were acting in a caring capacity.

Research

The Act clarifies that people lacking capacity may be involved in research projects if they agree to the research, if a carer agrees they would have wanted to be part of the research, if the research will directly benefit them, or if it will not, that it could not be carried out with people who had capacity.

Terms likely to be encountered by professionals

Independent mental capacity advocates (IMCAs)

These are individuals appointed by the court to speak for someone who lacks capacity but has no-one to speak for them. They may challenge a clinician or carer, and represent the person's wishes and feelings, though their decisions are not legally binding, only to be considered.

Lasting power of attorney

LPA replaced enduring power of attorney (EPA) but conveys similar powers. The LPA persists after capacity is lost and cannot then be revoked. A key difference is that it now applies to healthcare decisions as well as financial decisions.

Deputies

The Court of Protection may appoint deputies (these replace the old system of receiverships) who can make decisions about financial, health, and social care. They cannot refuse life-saving treatment. Deputies will only be appointed if recurrent decisions are likely, so the court cannot rule as a one-off.

Reference

1. Mental Capacity Act 2005 http://www.justice.gov.uk/guidance/mental-capacity.htm

Mental health legislation

- Most countries have some form of mental health legislation. The purpose of such legislation is to provide protections from harm for people with mental disorders, to protect others from the effects of mental disorder, to protect people with mental disorder, a vulnerable group, from mistreatment and excessive detention, and in some cases, to assist in the care of people unable by reason of mental disorder to make informed decisions about healthcare.
- In the UK, formal legislation has been available since the early nineteenth century. For any legislation, common themes are likely to be some definition of mental disorder, specification of grounds for detention and compulsory treatment, clear legal redress including grounds for appeal, and provision for scrutiny of the application of the law. There is often confusion around when mental health law should be applied and when considerations of capacity issues apply; practice varies between countries.

Mental Health Act 1983

In England and Wales, the Mental Health Act 1983 applies; a newer act (2007) provides some amendments. The main sections encountered in clinical practice include:

- ***Section 5(4):*** nurse holding powers—power of nurses to hold a patient for up to 6 h until a doctor arrives.
- ***Section 5(2):*** power of a doctor to detain a patient in a hospital for up to 72 h because of mental disorder; decision on further detention must be made in this time.
- ***Section 2:*** power of three professionals to detain a person with mental disorder in a hospital for up to 28 days for assessment.
- ***Section 3:*** power of three professionals to detain a person with mental disorder in a hospital for up to 6 months for treatment of the mental disorder.

In Scotland and Northern Ireland, there is independent legislation which largely follows the same principles as England and Wales. Scottish law already provides for limited community treatment orders. Northern Irish law allows initial detention periods of up to 7 days, followed by treatment up to 6 months. In the Republic of Ireland, the Mental Health Act 2001 allowed certain people including doctors and police officers to detain a person in a psychiatric hospital for a short period before a consultant psychiatrist applied to extend the period of detention.

Mental Health Act 2007

A new mental health bill was proposed for some years for England and Wales. Extensive consultation has led to substantial amendments. The bill became law in 2007; the principal changes include:

- Introduction of limited community treatment orders.
- Simplifying the definition of mental disorder.
- Changing the definition of treatability.
- Broadening the range of professionals allowed to make decisions about detention.
- Making appeals compulsory after long periods of detention.

Mental Health Act—in-patient issues

Likely issues in a general hospital

Among older general hospital in-patients, the MHA may occasionally be used to assist with patients who are delirious and require administration of calming medication and prevention from leaving the ward. Physicians may sometimes erroneously request that in-patients with a mental disorder (usually dementia) be detained to allow treatment of a physical illness which they cannot consent to. Among older psychiatric in-patients, people with dementia may initially consent to admission but need regular restraint to prevent them leaving. People with depression may deteriorate to the point that ECT is required but is either refused or capacity is absent.

Scenario 1

A 73-year-old woman is an in-patient with peripheral vascular disease. She has established moderate dementia and lives in a care home. She requires a below-knee amputation of the right lower limb or gangrene is likely, in the opinion of the vascular surgeon treating her. She refuses surgery but cannot give informed consent. A psychiatrist is asked to 'section' her. The psychiatrist writes: 'This woman has established Alzheimer's disease of moderate severity. She lacks capacity to give informed consent and there is no prospect of this being recovered. She refuses the surgery on the grounds of not wanting an operation. The Mental Health Act cannot be used to treat a physical condition, unless that condition is clearly the cause of her mental disorder (dementia). It is up to the treating team to decide whether this operation is in the best interests of this patient, after consulting with family in usual way.'

Scenario 2

A 65-year-old man was admitted to a medical ward with an overdose of 35 paracetamol tablets. He agreed to transfer to a psychiatric unit for assessment on a Friday night, once medically fit. On Sunday morning he states 'I am going home'. He has severe osteoarthritis and an alcohol problem, and has been depressed for 3 months since his wife died. He won't answer questions about whether he will do this again. A duty doctor writes in his notes: 'This man appears clinically depressed and took a substantial recent overdose. He is now medically fit to leave general hospital. His suicide risk is high and I am detaining him on section 5(2) of the Mental Health Act to allow further assessment, pending consultant review tomorrow morning.'

Mental Health Act—community issues

Among older psychiatric patients in the community, common issues involve patients with dementia who neglect themselves, refuse social care, or refuse to enter a care home. As with younger people, older people with serious mental illness including depressive illness, mania, and schizophrenia may refuse services/treatment and represent a high risk, needing compulsory admission. Some older people have physical frailty which may increase the urgency of assessment, e.g. patients with congestive cardiac failure may refuse diuretics when depressed, putting themselves at risk.

Scenario 1

A 81-year-old man has a history of recurrent depressive disorder and now mild dementia. He is followed up by a community mental health team. In recent months he has become low in mood, apathetic, eats poorly, and fails to take antidepressant and antihypertensive medication regularly. His wife is now very worried as he is eating poorly, losing weight, and not drinking enough fluid. When seen by the community team he states 'there is no point to treatment; I don't deserve it. They are better off without me.' His community nurse contacts medical and social work colleagues to request a Mental Health Act assessment: 'This man is deteriorating quickly and neither myself nor his wife can get him to eat or drink. I believe he is at risk of renal failure and we cannot get medication in reliably. I have no choice but to request urgent Mental Health Act assessment.'

Scenario 2

A 77-year-old woman is referred to a psychiatrist by her GP. She has had no previous physical or mental health problems but her daughter reports she has been very suspicious about the neighbours recently and thinks her food may be poisoned. She tells the psychiatrist that new neighbours are pumping gas in to her home and contaminating her water supplies. She hears them 'interfering with the plumbing at night'. She adamantly refuses treatment 'there is nothing wrong with me'. She is terrified of admission to 'the loony bin'. The psychiatrist writes: 'The diagnosis is of late-onset schizophrenia and the symptoms are typical. There is no evidence of dementia. She is adamantly opposed to treatment. In theory she could be detained and treated with antipsychotic medication in hospital but I do not think we should do this as: 1. the response rate to such treatment is modest; 2. she is able to lead a reasonable quality of life despite her symptoms; 3. she would be extremely upset by forcible admission to hospital; 4. there is very low risk of her acting forcibly against the neighbour, other than complaints. We will follow her up through our community team in case of deterioration.'

End-of-life issues

Palliative care

[illegible]

Where people die

[illegible]

Psychological support for the dying

[illegible]

To feed or not to feed

[illegible]

End-of-life issues

Palliative care

This term 'palliative care'[1] refers to care which is holistic, i.e. offers care for the body, mind, and spirit and which is not primarily directed towards cure. It is given to patients in whom death is expected in the near future and key goals including preparing the patient and family for the death and making the most of the time left. Specific services have been set up in many countries to provide such care. In the UK they are known as palliative care teams and are best known for dealing with terminal stages of cancer in both young and old, and management of progressive neurological conditions like motor neuron disease. There is increased interest in how the palliative care model may help people with dementia. Dementia of whatever cause is usually progressive and fatal. Mean time from diagnosis to death in dementia is 5–8 years. Some organizations deliver palliative care to people/families with dementia, e.g. Admiral Nurses in the UK, who are specialist dementia nurses with a role supporting the family and carers of people with dementia.

Where people die

Clear trends can be seen in location of death for older people. As the populations of Western countries age, increasing proportions live in residential and nursing homes. In the last two decades, there has been a significant fall in the proportion of older people in the UK dying at home (now about a quarter) with increases in those dying in hospital (over half) and in care homes (a sixth). US research also shows that the place of death of those with dementia is much more likely to be a care home (67%) than for those with cancer. Individual choice should be accommodated if possible; many older people will be surprisingly keen on dying in an institutional setting, it seems the presence of loved ones, and not being a burden, may outweigh any wishes to die in their own homes.

Psychological care of the dying

The majority of older people probably die a good death, i.e. without evidence of distressing pain or other physical discomfort and without severe psychological distress. Older people who are dying may undergo anticipatory changes in preparation for death which resemble a grief reaction, including disbelief, shock and bewilderment, bargaining, depression, and resolution. In dementia, realization of impending death may be absent. For relatives, anticipatory grief is common. The family may have been robbed of the person they knew by the dementia so rehearsing and undergoing grieving during life is understandable and may allow easier coping with death itself. It is unusual to have to use specific psychiatric skills with families, other than sympathy, listening, and answering questions.

To feed or not to feed?

In the last 20 years, nutritional support in the form of enteral feeding has become widely available. The most common intervention is nasogastric tube feeding, but PEG tubes are also available. PEG tubes are usually considered for medium- to longer-term feeding in those unlikely to recover the ability to eat due to dysphagia. Complications of PEG tubes include gastrointestinal tract perforation, bleeding, inhalation, infection, and consequences of sedation. The procedure is sometimes proposed for people with dementia who are losing weight due to dementia. Several hundred such procedures are carried out per year in the UK. This raises important clinical and ethical issues:

- It is widely held that PEG tubing removes the risk of inhalation pneumonias—this is untrue and the rate of such infections is unchanged after PEG.
- PEG tubing in dementia has been shown not to improve quality of life, infection rate, bedsores, or survival.
- While withholding nutrition is legally counted the same as removing treatment, there is no obligation to introduce treatments which are futile, i.e. cannot lead to a meaningful improvement in quality of life.

Reference

1. Hughes JC, Jolley D, Jordan A, Sampson EL. Palliative care in dementia: Issues and evidence. Adv Psychiat Treatment. 2007;13:251–60.See also: General Medical Council ☞ http://www.gmc-uk.org/

Elder abuse

Elder abuse is the term most often used to describe maltreatment of older people. Many acts of commission or omission can lead to harm for an older person. Technically, abuse refers to an act of commission causing harm, e.g. stealing, punching, shouting at, or sexually assaulting a victim. Neglect refers to an act of omission which leads to harm; examples may be withholding food or ignoring cries for help. We will use the term 'abuse' to cover all such acts. Abuse may also be thought of as emotional, verbal, humiliation, financial, violent, or sexual, or oversedation, restraint, or omission of care. There is greatly increased interest in the area, partly due to older people's advocacy groups, partly because of public awareness of the scale of the problem. It has been estimated that at least 2 million older people in the USA (population 340 million) and 500,000 older people in the UK (population 67 million) experience significant abuse per year. Estimates of the true scale of the problem often depend on proxy measures such as helpline reports or selective surveys, and depend greatly on the definition of abuse. The reliability of reports of people with memory problems may be called into question.

Always abuse

- Violence including hitting, pushing, kicking.
- Sexual assault.
- Financial abuse including stealing, forging cheques.
- Deliberate omission of provision of food, warmth, medical care.

Often abuse

- Bed sores.
- Oversedation with psychoactive drugs.
- Restraint.
- Restriction of food/access to money/privacy.
- Altering of will in favour of new person.

Where does abuse occur?

- Action on Elder Abuse estimate (2004 figures) that 67% of abuse takes place in the older person's home, 5% in hospitals, and 22% in residential or nursing homes.
- In care homes, yearly prevalence of abuse reported as 6–10% physical abuse, 11–40% psychological abuse.
- Among community carers of people with dementia, 5–47% yearly prevalence figures are reported for violence against a person with dementia.
- Rates of violence against carers by people with dementia are estimated at close to 100% in residential homes, i.e. professional carers in these settings endure regular physical aggression.

Types of abuse

Financial abuse

This may take many forms. Direct stealing of money by a carer or local youth, failing to return change when shopping is done as a service, use of an older person's bank card, excessive pressure on older people to sign to a poorly understood financial commitment, signing cheques on the account of an older person for personal use may all be seen. More subtly, a new carer may influence an older person to alter the terms of a will in his/her favour. In some cases, this may be disputed by family, and judgements of the capacity of the person with dementia to make a will (testamentary capacity) may be required. Prosecution is often difficult due to lack of reliable evidence. The new MCA, 2005, enacted in England and Wales in 2007, provides for protection in this area: as before, people may donate power of attorney over financial matters (now known as lasting power of attorney), the court of protection may appoint deputies to manage financial affairs for an incapacitated person, and a specific criminal offence of ill-treatment or neglect of a person who lacks capacity has been introduced.

Sexual abuse

The prevalence of sexual abuse of older people is unknown, but represents under 10% of cases of elder abuse. Serious sexual assaults are less common than on younger people; serious offenders against older people are likely to have significant psychological disturbance and may be incarcerated for long periods for treatment and public safety. Signs of sexual abuse may include unexplained sexual disease or anal/vaginal bleeding and bruising.

Physical abuse

Including all forms of physical abuse, violence between older people, especially those with dementia, and their carers, is common. In specialist care home settings, assault of staff by patients is commonplace, often daily. Physical abuse of residents by staff is reported in up to 10% of residents per year in care homes and up to 50% in community settings. The distinction between self-protection and violence, and the status of use of gentle force in ensuring personal care, is often a matter of judgement.

Approach to possible cases of abuse

- Get a clear history.
- Decide if local safeguarding adults procedures should be invoked.
- Establish capacity of victim to participate in decision-making.
- Establish carer characteristics and account of events.
- Get specific expertise if needed, e.g. financial advocate, solicitor, police.
- Arrange a multidisciplinary case conference.
- Consider help required by carer—treatment, psychological assessment, relief from care burden.
- Decide if legal proceedings are needed.
- Protect both parties by establishing third-party support, e.g. independent deputy appointed by court of protection.
- Relocate vulnerable person, e.g. to new care home, if appropriate.

Case example

Mrs R is an 84-year-old woman with a 3-year history of AD. She lives alone and is cared for by a 50-year-old unmarried son who has a history of alcohol abuse. Neighbours express a concern that she is losing weight, her clothes are not being changed, and her medications are being given chaotically. The son permits carers only to give a meal daily and give medication. She later has bruises that both he and she explain are due to a fall. He refuses help for his alcohol use and won't allow her to have a respite admission to a care home. She says she is 'not bothered' and wants to stay at home. A multidisciplinary safeguarding case conference is held, led by social services. The son, her case worker from social services, a police officer, a neighbour, a manager of the care agency, and an old age psychiatrist who has seen her on four occasions are present. The GP has sent a report expressing her concern about well-being. The outcome is that a letter is sent to him stating that he must allow two carers access to his mother three times a day and a respite admission to a care home each 8 weeks. Legal proceedings to take his mother into care will be started if he does not comply. The social worker obtains all eligible financial benefits to offset the costs of the extra care and he is offered help from the community alcohol team. No criminal charges are brought.

Crime and older people

Older people and offending

- Older people in the UK represent under 1% of all those convicted of an offence.
- The number of older people convicted of an offence is rising.
- The prison population of those over 60 years is rising.
- A tenth of convictions among older people are for sexual offences.

Psychiatric disorder and crime in older people

- Among convicted people, rates of psychiatric disorder are very low.
- Most assaults by people with dementia are unreported.
- There is no evidence that paranoid illness, mood disorder, or dementia increase the risk of offending among older people.
- Alcohol may precipitate offending in older people.
- Drug-related crime is very rare.
- Abnormal personality traits are found less frequently among older offenders than among younger offenders.

The older psychiatric patient in court

Most countries will seek to divert older people from the criminal justice system. In particular, people with dementia who lack criminal responsibility or fitness to plead are unlikely to recover it with treatment and are unlikely to come to trial. Alternative disposals to prison may include care homes, probation, or psychiatric hospitalization.

Checklist in establishing fitness to plead in the UK (equivalent to 'competence to stand trial' in the USA)

Can the person:

- Understand the charge they are answering?
- Understand what entering a plea means?
- Understand the consequences of a guilty and a not guilty plea?
- Follow evidence?
- Challenge proceedings?
- Challenge a juror?
- Instruct a lawyer?

Older people as victims of crime

Older people are much less likely to be a victim of crime than younger people. In particular, they are much less likely to be a victim of violent crime. It is widely held that fear of crime is higher among older people but the best evidence does not support this, showing older people to have a realistic appraisal of risk. Some older people lose confidence and may become housebound or even institutionalized after becoming a victim of crime. This is more likely among women and the socially isolated.

Prescribing issues in older people

Pharmacokinetics

Pharmacokinetics is the study of the metabolism and action of drugs, with particular emphasis on time required for absorption, duration of action, distribution in the body, and method of excretion. The ageing process can bring about changes in the following pharmacokinetic parameters:

Absorption

The absorption of drugs may be slowed down or delayed in older people due to a number of factors including reduction in gastric pH, decrease of the size of the intestinal absorption area, and reduced blood flow to the digestive system due to an overall decrease in cardiac output. All these factors can contribute to an overall decreased bioavailability of drugs in older people.

Distribution

The distribution of drugs is influenced by the composition of the body. In older people, a number of changes in body composition could influence drug distribution. An increased proportion of fat tissue in older people can increase the volume of distribution of drugs, and as most psychotropic medications are stored in fat tissue, their elimination half-life is consequently increased. A decrease in the lean body mass and water content can result in higher concentrations of drugs such as alcohol that are distributed throughout the body fluids. A decrease in the overall albumin concentration can result in high concentration of free (not bound with plasma proteins) levels of drug, thus resulting in high levels of drugs crossing the blood–brain barrier and producing more side effects. In some cases, a decrease in cerebral blood flow may result in decreased levels of drugs in the brain.

Metabolism

Most psychotropic drugs are metabolized in the liver, with the notable exception of lithium which is renally excreted. Hepatic blood flow is known to decrease with age thus increasing the elimination half-life of drugs metabolized in the liver. As a consequence, a prolongation of action after a single dose and delayed accumulation on multiple doses can be seen in older people.

Excretion

A reduction in renal function is common in advanced age. Average renal excretion declines by a third from youth to old age. Individual older people may have perfectly normal excretion, but some, especially those with concomitant physical illness, may have difficulties with water-soluble drugs such as lithium. Guidelines for lithium prescription recommend using a single bedtime dosing regimen, regular monitoring of blood lithium levels and renal function, and dose adjustments according to declining renal function.

Pharmacodynamics

- Pharmacodynamics deals with the mechanisms by which drugs exert their actions on the body. In other words, it is the study of how drugs act at target sites of action in the body. A number of pharmacodynamic changes in old age tend to alter sensitivity to drugs, even when plasma concentrations are similar to those in younger people.
- The elderly are particularly sensitive to sedatives, antiparkinsonian drugs, and drugs with anticholinergic properties (Table 9.1). Ageing brain cells are more vulnerable to the excitotoxicity caused by glutamate overactivity. Age-associated changes in the brain result in general changes in cellular metabolism. These result in deficits in dopamine, acetylcholine, serotonin, and noradrenaline neurotransmitter systems resulting in diminished efficiency of homeostatic mechanisms in the ageing brain. Any direct influence of ageing itself on drug binding at individual receptors, and subsequent post-synaptic effects, is poorly understood.
- The above-mentioned factors contribute to a reduction in normal regulatory processes within the brain and make it more vulnerable to develop severe reactions with drugs. It is probable that the majority of adverse reactions to drugs which are common among older people are related to the presence of physical illness, and increased prescribing, rather than to pharmacodynamic changes *per se*.

Table 9.1 Pharmacodynamic factors in the ageing brain

Neurotransmitter	Age changes	Consequences
GABA system	Receptor changes Declining mitochondrial function	Increased susceptibility to sedatives, e.g. benzodiazepines
Dopamine system	Decreased dopamine production Decreased number of neurons in nigro-striatal system	Increased susceptibility to drug-induced parkinsonism
Acetylcholine system	Cortical degeneration Decreased nicotine affinity Decreased acetylcholine production	Increased risk of delirium Increased susceptibility to anticholinergic drugs
Noradrenaline system	Degeneration of locus coeruleus Depletion of noradrenaline Compensatory activation of other noradrenergic neurons	Slowed cognition Sensitivity to yohimbine
Serotonin system	Reduction in 5HT2 receptors Reduction in serotonin uptake sites	Decreased effectiveness of serotonergic drugs, e.g. SSRIs
Glutamate system	Decreased NMDA receptors Impairment of cellular energy metabolism	Cognitive decline Neurotoxicity

Polypharmacy

- The incidence of both psychiatric disorders and medical illnesses is higher among older people. These conditions frequently occur simultaneously and are often chronic, lasting for the lifetime of the individual; consequently, older patients often require more medications than younger people. Older people also tend to be higher consumers of over-the-counter drugs.
- A combination of use of multiple drugs for medical and psychiatric illness along with over-the-counter preparations and the pharmacokinetic and dynamic changes in the body makes older people vulnerable to a wide range of side effects. The dilemma faced by the physician is how to treat an illness without causing more harm than good. This is not helped by the fact that most research studies on the use and safety of drugs are conducted on younger people, and physicians caring for older people have to generalize those findings to their older patients.
- These problems can result in a reluctance to prescribe or treat a problem. This can be positive, as it tends to encourage us to look for non-pharmacological methods of management in disorders such as BPSD or psychological interventions for depression and anxiety. It can, however, also lead to a delay in the alleviation of distress, leading to poor quality of life, and sometimes to increased risk.
- It is, therefore, important for physicians to realize that the response to treatment is generally good in older people with specific psychiatric disorders such as a major depressive episode, and that the risk of not treating or under-treating (low doses) can be greater than the potential risks of treatment. Although the choice of safest combination of medications would ultimately depend on the characteristics of the individual patient, the following strategies might be useful in avoiding harmful effects of polypharmacy:

Antidepressants

Tricyclic antidepressants:

- Tricyclics are not recommended as a first-line treatment of depression or mixed depression and anxiety states.
- Some patients may still be treated with tricyclics if they have been stable on them for many years or for other reasons, such as chronic pain and neuralgia.
- Their tendency to cause sedation and postural hypotension may increase the risk of falls and excessive sedation if combined with benzodiazepines and antipsychotics.
- Their combination with analgesics containing opioid derivatives such as cocodamol may cause/aggravate constipation.
- They invariably increase anticholinergic burden for older people, for example if used with trospium chloride in patients with bladder frequency.

SSRIs:

- Most SSRIs compete for the same metabolic pathway used by β-blockers, benzodiazepines, and some antiarrhythmics.
- SSRIs in combination with aspirin might increase a tendency to gastrointestinal bleeds/ulceration especially in very old (85+) patients.

MAOIs:

- A class of antidepressants rarely used nowadays due to dangerous interactions with opiate analgesics (especially pethidine), nasal decongestants (like pseudoephedrine), and other antidepressants (risk of hypertensive crisis) and tyramine-containing foods.
- Moclobemide is a safer modern alternative monoamine oxidase inhibitor (MAOI).

Antipsychotics

Conventional antipsychotics:

- Carry a high risk of causing movement disorders (see section *tardive dyskinesia* in chapter 6).
- Have a tendency to cause sedation and postural hypotension that in combination with other sedating drugs, such as benzodiazepines; tricyclic antidepressants and mirtazapine may increase the risk of falls.

Atypical antipsychotics:

- Recommended first-line treatment for psychotic symptoms.
- Olanzapine has a tendency to disturb glucose and lipid metabolism and can aggravate/disturb treatment of diabetic patients on oral hypoglycaemics and insulin.
- Quetiapine has a tendency to cause sedation and postural hypotension, which might increase the risk of falls in combination with other drugs with sedating side effects.
- Newer agents have been designed to minimize these side effects: lurasidone, lumateperone, cariprazine, olanzapine–samidorphan combination. These medications are rarely familiar to non-specialists.

Aggression in the elderly

Being asked to see an aggressive elderly patient is common, both in liaison and community settings. Aggression is usually seen in one of the following four clinical scenarios.

Aggression in dementia

In most cases the reasons for aggression cannot be explained by the patient nor do they have any memory of their aggressive behaviour. The episodes of aggression are unpredictable and occur impulsively. The usual scenario is of a patient becoming physically or verbally aggressive while receiving care from staff or relatives, for example in personal hygiene. The patient can often simply be distracted from the target of aggression. This type of aggressive behaviour can be persistent and cause a strain on carers. It is one of the commonest reasons for placement in nursing homes for patients with dementia. It is among the commonest reasons for clinicians to be asked to prescribe for people with dementia.

Aggression in delirium

The aggressive behaviour, either physical or verbal, appears to be random and unpredictable. The course is fluctuating and as in dementia, patients appear to be more disturbed and aggressive at night-time. The aggressive behaviour may be in response to delusions or hallucinations combined with the disorientation caused by an alien environment if the patient is in hospital.

Aggression in delirium can put the patient at risk of harm to themselves due to lack of cooperation with the staff in taking medication and accepting care, failure to eat and drink adequately, and exposure to extremes of weather.

Aggression in depression

This type of aggression usually occurs in the setting of irritability. Patients are usually aware of their irritability and may be angry with themselves and want to be left alone. Irritability/agitation/aggression in depression has to be taken seriously, requiring a detailed risk assessment of harm to self or others.

Aggression in psychosis/paranoid patients

Here the aggression usually occurs in response to the patient's delusional beliefs and perceptual abnormalities, such as auditory hallucinations. Most patients with psychotic illness will never be violent. The patient usually expresses reasons for being aggressive, is likely to have a good recollection of the aggressive episodes, and may express remorse/guilt afterwards. It is important to recognize that the patient may be aggressive as a defence against profound fear and insecurity. Aggression with psychosis warrants a detailed risk assessment of harm to self or others and not just prescription of antipsychotic medication. Antipsychotic medication may rapidly induce sedation as a side effect, but its core antipsychotic effect will typically take at least a week.

Assessing aggressive patients

- Management of all aggressive patients should involve a thorough assessment and not just prescription of psychotropic medications.
- Aggressive patients are vulnerable to self-harm, harm to others, neglect, abuse, and inappropriate placements for future care.

Assessment

A comprehensive assessment of an aggressive patient should include the following:

- A detailed history of the aggressive behaviour is extremely important as aggression is a loose term and can have different meanings for people from different professional backgrounds.
- One of the useful ways of assessing episodes of aggression could be by dividing each episode into antecedents, behaviour, and consequences (the so-called ABC approach). With this simple approach, each episode of aggression can be analysed with useful information about the possible causes/provocations of aggressive behaviour, the actual nature of the behaviour (verbal/physical aggression and its severity), and the consequences of that behaviour(i.e. is it putting the patient or carers at risk of harm? Is it resulting in isolation/neglect of the patient? Is the behaviour reinforced by attention or by failure to challenge the patient?) The 'ABC technique' is especially helpful in specialist dementia care homes.
- A detailed history of present and past illness, looking at the pattern of aggression (acute or chronic), symptoms of associated psychiatric disorders (depression, dementia, psychosis), and past history of mental disorders.
- A detailed mental state examination, including cognitive assessment is key to the management plan as it will pick up signs and symptoms of associated psychiatric disorders.
- A list of baseline laboratory investigations (mid-stream specimen of urine (MSU), blood counts, and metabolic profile) can be useful to help rule out delirium or associated medical problems. An example of an underlying medical problem causing episodes of aggression/agitation would be a diabetic patient becoming aggressive during episodes of hypoglycaemia.

Case example

An 89-year-old woman with established dementia lives in a care home. She requires near total care. In recent weeks, she has become aggressive to the care staff when they attempt to bathe or dress her. The GP prescribes risperidone 0.5 mg twice daily. Carers report her to be calmer but less verbally able and no longer walking. A community psychiatric nurse (CPN) is called and visits. Her report states: 'The patient has painful arthritic hands which need improved analgesia.' On tramadol, she is in far less pain and is not constipated. Risperidone is successfully removed and she is more alert. A senior care assistant assists junior staff with personal care.

Specific management of aggression

Pharmacological management

Use of psychotropic medication should only be considered as one component of the management plan for the individual patient, keeping in mind that fact that these drugs tend to be frequently overused and can cause a number of serious side effects. Rating scales to quantify symptoms include the Cohen–Mansfield Agitation Inventory (CMAI).

Antipsychotic medication

Antipsychotics are the drug of choice for aggression associated with psychosis, although they can also be effective in treating aggression/agitation in delirium and dementia. They are least effective in treating behavioural disturbances such as wandering, excessive vocalization, and sexual disinhibition. The atypical antipsychotics such as risperidone and olanzapine and, amongst typicals, haloperidol are most commonly used due to their high potency and low dose requirement. In addition, brexpiprazole has received US Food and Drug Administration (FDA) supplemental approval for treating agitation in the context of Alzheimer's disease. In general, the lowest dose possible of antipsychotic should be used and treatment should be time limited.

Antidepressants

These can be used in aggressive patients with an underlying depression. SSRIs such as citalopram are drugs of first choice due to their better side-effect profile. The usefulness of antidepressants such as trazodone has also been reported in aggressive patients with dementia where there is a possibility of underlying depression (limited data).

Benzodiazepines

Short-acting benzodiazepines such as lorazepam (e.g. start with a low dose 0.5–1 mg) can be useful in controlling acute episodes of aggression in conjunction with antipsychotics or on their own when there is a medical reason for not prescribing antipsychotics. Their long-term use, however, is not recommended. There are no controlled trial data to support this strategy so their effectiveness beyond short-term calming has not been established.

Non-pharmacological interventions

- These are planned and tailored according to the needs of the individual patient keeping in mind the underlying diagnosis, the nature of the aggression, and the associated risk of harm to self and others.
- Environmental influences and the nature of relationships with carers are important considerations in managing aggression. The first step in this process is to decide whether the current environment is safe for the patient and if not, what would be the most suitable environment for them to be managed. For instance, some psychotic or depressed patients might require management in an acute in-patient facility.

- For aggressive patients with underlying dementia, it is useful to assess whether the current environment and skills of the carers are adequate to manage their difficult behaviour or whether they require in-patient management in hospital and discharge to a care facility with a more suitable environment and staff to deal with their behavioural difficulties.
- For dementia patients with a tendency to aggression, simple techniques like regular orientation in their environment, and a step-by-step approach with explanation when providing personal care such as changing clothes and bathing, are appropriate as a first-level intervention. Familiar nursing staff that can form a relationship with the patient and have knowledge of their background help in dealing with most patients with mild to moderate levels of aggression.

See figure 9.1 for a suggested approach to managing aggression.

Aggression Reported

Background information gathering:

- Nature of Aggression: verbal/physical/frequency
- History of mental illness: mood disorder/psychosis/dementia/drug abuse
- History of physical illness: pain/constipation/head injury
- Setting: home/care home/general hospital
- Onset: acute/chronic

Mental and Cognitive State Examination

No mental illness	Mood disorders	Psychosis	Dementia	Delirium
• Consider possibility of abuse **Yes**: *Report to:* • Police • Local authority **No**: *Report to:* • Referring authority	• Assess suicide risk • Consider hospital admission • Consider use of MHA*/ admission against will • Antipsychotics • Antidepressants	• Assess risk of harm • Consider hospital admission • Consider use of MHA*/ admission against will • Consider environmental causes & poss. changes • Antipsychotics	• Assess risk of abuse • Consider environmental causes & poss. changes • ABC** technique to plan management • Antipsychotics • Antidepressants	• Baseline investigations • Consider admission in general hospital • Antibiotics • Antipsychotics • Benzodiazepines

* Mental Health Act

** Antecedents, Behaviours and Consequences

Fig 9.1 Management of aggression

Sleep disorders/insomnia

Sleep disturbance in the elderly can be caused by a number of factors acting in isolation or in combination. It includes physiological changes associated with ageing, poor sleep hygiene, medical illnesses, and adverse effects of medications. It may be secondary or primary sleep disorders. Secondary sleep disorders may result from psychiatric conditions such as depression, anxiety, and dementia. Primary sleep disorders include sleep apnoea, REM sleep behaviour disorder, and primary insomnia. Sleep problems are exceptionally common in Alzheimer's disease, and [illegible] such as Parkinson's [illegible].

The International Classification of Sleep Disorders divides sleep disorders into seven categories:

1. Insomnia
2. Sleep-related breathing disorders (e.g. obstructive sleep apnoea)
3. Central disorders of hypersomnolence (e.g. narcolepsy)
4. Circadian rhythm sleep–wake disorders
5. Parasomnias (e.g. REM sleep behaviour disorder, [illegible]; differential diagnosis includes frontal seizures)
6. Sleep-related movement disorders (e.g. restless legs syndrome, periodic limb movement disorder)
7. Other sleep disorders

Treatment of insomnia

- A [illegible] large number of elderly people are prescribed sedative hypnotics. A number of studies have [illegible] in the UK and [illegible] elderly people are prescribed [illegible] benzodiazepines [illegible] falls [illegible] to look at all possible causes of sleep disturbance before prescribing hypnotics.
- Excessive time in bed, irregular sleep times, [illegible] and excessive intake of stimulants such as caffeine [illegible] are common causes for poor sleep hygiene [illegible].
- It is also important to [illegible] that adequate exposure to [illegible] light decreases with advancing age [illegible].
- Sleep disturbance caused by [illegible] is one of the common [illegible].
- Bladder problems resulting in [illegible] are [illegible] falls and [illegible].
- Patients with [illegible] may respond better to [illegible].

Sleep disorders/insomnia

Sleep disturbance in the elderly can be caused by a number of factors acting in isolation or in combination such as physiological changes associated with ageing, poor sleep, hygiene, medical illnesses, and psychiatric conditions causing secondary or primary sleep disorders. Secondary sleep disorders may result from psychiatric conditions such as depression, anxiety, and dementia. Primary sleep disorders include sleep apnoea, REM sleep behaviour disorder, and primary insomnia. Sleep disorders are common in Alzheimer's disease[1], and parasomnias in synucleinopathies such as Parkinson's disease.

The International Classification of Sleep Disorders divides sleep disorders into seven categories[2]:

1. Insomnia
2. Sleep-related breathing disorders (e.g. obstructive sleep apnoea)
3. Central disorders of hypersomnolence (e.g. narcolepsy)
4. Circadian rhythm sleep–wake disorders
5. Parasomnias (e.g. REM sleep behaviour disorder, REM sleep without atonia—related to Lewy Body Dementia; differential diagnosis includes frontal seizures)
6. Sleep-related movement disorders (Restless Legs Syndrome, periodic limb movement disorder)
7. Other sleep disorders

Treatment of insomnia

- A disproportionately large number of elderly people are prescribed sedative hypnotics. A number of studies have shown that in the UK and North America between 5% and 33% of elderly people are prescribed hypnotics for sleep problems. Benzodiazepines or benzodiazepine receptor agonists are the most commonly used drugs. These drugs are associated with increased risk of ataxia, falls, and memory impairment, which become more important in the very old age group. It is important to look at all possible causes of sleep disturbance before prescribing hypnotics.
- Excessive time in bed with regular sleeping hours, noisy environments, lack of exercise, and excessive intake of stimulants such as caffeine are all common causes for poor sleep hygiene and can be easily altered without prescription of hypnotics.
- It is also important to assess the total amount of sleep in 24 hours as sleep requirement decreases with advancing age and some older people tend to take afternoon naps that reduce the sleep requirement at night-time.
- Sleep disturbance caused by pain—especially due to musculoskeletal disorders—is one of the common causes of insomnia and can easily be treated with a bedtime dose of NSAID medication.
- Bladder problems resulting in nocturia commonly contribute to sleep disturbance, falls, and hip fractures. When present, nocturia should prompt investigations for diabetes, prostate disease in men, and bladder prolapse in women.
- Patients with obstructive lung disease can present with sleep disturbance and may respond better to the use of long-acting beta-agonists that minimize disruptive nocturnal dyspnoea.

- GI reflux can cause sleep disturbance and, if present, requires dietary counselling and the use of a proton pump inhibitor.
- Chronic congestive cardiac failure can also present with sleep disturbance and its aggressive treatment to prevent nocturnal dyspnoea and orthopnoea can enhance sleep quality.
- Depressed patients with marked sleep disturbance can be treated with sedating antidepressants such as mirtazapine or trazodone.
- Patients with dementia having sleep disturbance usually require a combination of behavioural and environmental measures such as reassurance, late day limitation of external stimulation, familiar and restful environments, along with hypnotic medication. As dementia advances, loss of normal sleep–wake cycle is common and treatment to induce sleep may only benefit carers rather than patients.

Rapid eye movement sleep behaviour disorder

Rapid eye movement sleep behaviour disorder (RBD) is often encountered in patients diagnosed with Parkinson's disease dementia or dementia with Lewy bodies. Patients lose normal atonia during REM sleep and can enact their dreams[3]. The differential diagnosis includes frontal seizures. Polysomnography can be used to confirm the diagnosis, but it may be evident clinically. Management options include clonazepam (e.g. 0.25 mg), immediate release melatonin, rivastigmine or pramipexole[4]. The bedroom should be made safe in case of night-time movements secondary to dream enactment. RBD can be secondary to antidepressants, particularly SSRIs, so the patient's other medications should be reviewed.

Basic principles of good sleep hygiene

Active measures to improve sleep:

- Use the bedroom only for sleep.
- Go to bed at a regular time every day.
- Make the bedroom calm, quiet, and protected from noise.
- Make the bed as comfortable as possible.
- Regular daytime exercise.
- Warm baths, soft music, and meditation help with relaxation before going to bed.
- Food including warm milk and carbohydrates can help with sleep.

Things to avoid for improving sleep:

- Napping during the daytime/afternoon.
- Going to bed early in the evening.
- Avoid stimulating drinks (tea, coffee, cola) before going to bed.
- Avoid smoking and alcohol consumption before going to bed.
- Heavy eating.
- Active exercise before bed time.
- Stimulating thoughts/problem solving while in bed.

Further reading

Howell M, Avidan AY, Foldvary-Schaefer N, et al. Management of REM sleep behavior disorder: An American Academy of Sleep Medicine clinical practice guideline. JCSM. 2023;19(4):759–768.

Prescribing for insomnia

- In primary insomnia, benzodiazepines have historically been the most commonly used hypnotics in older people (Table 9.2). They can be roughly divided into three groups; long acting, intermediate acting, and short acting, according to their half-lives. They decrease sleep latency and nocturnal awakening but should be used with caution as older people with advancing age become more sensitive to the effects of benzodiazepines. In some cases, they can cause amnesia, night-time wandering, and paradoxical agitation. Improved sleep may not justify the increased risk in older people, especially if they have additional risk factors for cognitive deterioration and falls.
- As a general principle, for sleep onset problems, a short-acting agent such as lorazepam or oxazepam may be effective. There have, however, been case reports of confusion, amnesia, and behaviour problems with these agents. In patients with early morning wakefulness an intermediate agent such as temazepam may be more useful.

Table 9.2 Hypnotics

Drug	Recommended daily dose for older people
Benzodiazepines	
Short acting	
Lorazepam	0.5–1 mg
Oxazepam	15–30 mg
Intermediate acting	
Nitrazepam	2.5–5 mg
Temazepam	10 mg
Long acting	
Chlordiazepoxide	5 mg
Clonazepam	0.25–0.5 mg
Diazepam	2–5 mg
Flurazepam	15 mg
Z-drugs	
Zopiclone	3.75–7.5 mg
Zaleplon	5 mg
Zolpidem	5 mg
Dual orexin receptor antagonists (DORAs)	
Daridorexant	25–50 mg
Suvorexant	10–20 mg
Lemborexant	5–10 mg
Melatonin agonists	
Ramelteon	8 mg

Long-acting benzodiazepines such as diazepam, flurazepam, and chlordiazepoxide are not recommended for insomnia in older patients. Clonazepam is recommended for RBD.

- The gamma-aminobutyric acid (GABA)-positive allosteric modulators (PAMs) ('z-drugs') have been shown to be effective in short-term treatment of insomnia and they have overtaken benzodiazepines as first-line agents. They have a relatively short half-life and are less likely to cause daytime sedation. They have an added advantage of lesser impairment of psychomotor and cognitive performance as compared with benzodiazepines. They have also been shown to be less disruptive of the normal sleep pattern. Commonly used non-benzodiazepine agents include zolpidem, zaleplon, and zopiclone.
- Dual orexin receptor antagonists (DORAs): these drugs block the action of orexins, which support wakefulness. There is some evidence that daridorexant can improve daytime functioning[5].
- The melatonin agonist ramelteon can be considered for sleep onset insomnia[6].

Psychosis in Parkinson's disease

- About 10–15% of patients with Parkinson's disease develop psychotic symptoms, of which visual hallucinations and persecutory delusions are the most common (also see section *BPSD in LBD* in Chapter 2). Treatment of psychosis associated with Parkinson's disease is challenging because a clinician is faced with what is described as the 'motion–emotion' conundrum. The dopaminergic drugs that improve movement are known to aggravate psychotic symptoms and, conversely, the use of antipsychotics aggravates the movement disorder.
- Clozapine and the new atypical antipsychotics have been the most commonly used drugs to treat these symptoms. Most early studies on treatment of psychosis in Parkinson's disease were done on clozapine and found it to be effective in ameliorating these symptoms. The recommended dose range is between 6.25 mg and 50 mg/day with most patients benefiting from a daily dose of 25 mg without having a negative impact on cognition. Clozapine carries a risk of causing agranulocytosis that increases with age and some patients might not be able to comply with the strict requirements of blood tests associated with the treatment.
- Other atypical antipsychotics with a lesser propensity to cause extrapyramidal side effects, including quetiapine, olanzapine, and risperidone, have been reported to be effective in lower doses. Quetiapine is a reasonable choice. Olanzapine in small doses (5 mg) has been reported to be effective in treating psychotic symptoms, but some patients may benefit from even lower doses of 2.5 mg. Risperidone may also be beneficial in lower doses and it is generally recommended that any of the three should be started at the lowest possible dose.
- Aripiprazole, an antipsychotic with a partial agonist action on dopamine D2 receptors, has been reported to be useful in psychotic symptoms associated with Parkinson's disease (small series). It has a lower likelihood of aggravating motor symptoms. It has the added advantage of being available in liquid form and can be started at a dose as low as 2.5 mg/day and then titrated up to 5 mg or 10 mg.
- Avoiding the problems with using dopamine blocking drugs, pimavanserin is licensed in the USA (not in the UK) for Parkinson's disease psychosis and works via inverse agonism at the 5-HT2A receptor. This means that it does not worsen motor symptoms. Dosage is 34 mg once daily without titration.

In psychosis in Parkinson's disease

- Review the patient's current dopaminergic medications and whether they have cognitive enhancers already in place or would benefit from starting one (e.g. rivastigmine).
- Pimavanserin (US) is the first drug approved for Parkinson's disease psychosis.
- Pimavanserin's mechanism of action is serotonergic and it does not have dopamine antagonist action, therefore not worsening motor symptoms.
- Clozapine has some controlled trial evidence of effectiveness for psychosis in Parkinson's disease.

- The risk of agranulocytosis limits the use of clozapine.
- Other atypical antipsychotics have less evidence of effectiveness and safety.
- Consider a second-generation antipsychotic like quetiapine.
- First-generation neuroleptics such as haloperidol and chlorpromazine should be avoided.

Further reading

An approach to managing psychosis in Parkinson's disease

Pirker W, Ferreira J, Rascol O et al. Management of Parkinson's disease psychosis—a European perspective. The Lancet Regional Health – Europe, 2026; 62.

Post-stroke depression

Psychiatric illness complicating the post-stroke period is common. The first 6 months after the stroke is considered a high-risk period for developing a psychiatric illness. Past and family history of psychiatric illness and a history of suicidal behaviour are important pointers. (Also see section on *vascular depression* in Chapter 4.)

Post-stroke depression

- A distinction from post-stroke emotionalism, a syndrome of dysregulation of emotional responses due to damage after stroke, should be made. Similar phenomena may be seen in other neurological disorders, e.g. motor neuron disease. On discussion of emotional issues, patients become emotional, crying easily, but can usually recover poise quickly. It is easily mistaken for depressive illness. SSRIs have been shown to reduce emotionalism after stroke, should this be distressing to the patient/carers.
- A number of reviews have reported the risk of post-stroke depression to be between 20% and 80%. A meta-analysis of 50 studies showed that prevalence of depression post stroke was 29%, with a recovery rate of 15–57% after 1 year (Ayerbe et al., 2013). The key predictors of developing post-stroke depression were stroke severity, disability, cognitive impairment, history of depression and anxiety (Ayerbe et al., 2013).
- Post-stroke patients are nearly twice as likely to develop major depression for up to 18 months after stroke as compared with the general population. It is important to recognize and aggressively treat post-stroke depression because it is associated with delayed functional recovery, decreased social function, and greater post-stroke mortality.
- In the literature, the usefulness of tricyclic antidepressants and SSRIs in post-stroke depression has been reported. There are fewer controlled trials conducted on other antidepressants such as venlafaxine and mirtazapine, but these are commonly used in clinical practice. SSRIs are recommended to be the first-line treatment in post-stroke depression because of better side-effect profile and less tendency to cause delirium and excessive sedation as compared with tricyclics.
- In the past some case reports had suggested that treatment with SSRIs might increase the risk of bleeding in some patients because of their effect on platelet function, but a major review conducted more recently did not report any causal relationship between the use of SSRIs and risk of bleeding after stroke.
- Among SSRIs there is little evidence to suggest the superiority of one over the other. As a general rule, treatment should be started at the lowest possible dose and increased gradually to higher doses with 1–2-week intervals. The recovery is expected to be slow and a trial of at least 6 weeks with a therapeutic dose is recommended before deciding whether the patient has responded to the treatment or not.
- If the patient responds, then the treatment should be continued for up to 12 months before deciding to gradually reduce the dose. If no clinical response is observed with treatment over 6 weeks or the medication is poorly tolerated, then the patient should be switched to a

different class of antidepressant. The most commonly used second-line antidepressants are mirtazapine and venlafaxine.

- In resistant cases where two trials of antidepressant medications fail, the mood deteriorates further, or the patient becomes suicidal, a psychiatric consultation should be immediately considered with the possibility of using ECT along with antidepressants (would be contraindicated in cases of recent intracerebral bleeding).

Post-stroke mania

- Post-stroke manic illness is rare but well recognized. Some patients can present with mixed symptoms of mania and depression with episodes of expansive or irritable mood, recklessness, over-talkativeness, and poor judgement. Past and family history of bipolar illness is important and all patients should be assessed for risk of suicide and aggression.
- A systematic review of 81 studies suggests that the clinical profile of post-stroke mania is similar to primary mania[7]. The most common symptom experienced first was euphoria and the typical patient was male and had a right-sided cerebral infarct, which is consistent with other evidence associating damage to the right orbitofrontal circuit, involved in mood regulation, to mania[7].
- These patients present with diagnostic and management challenges and should be referred for a psychiatric consultation. The treatment includes use of mood stabilizers with or without antipsychotic medication. There is no RCT evidence for managing post-stroke mania (also see section on *mania* in Chapter 4).
- Lithium should be used cautiously, especially if renal disease is present.
- Valproic acid is known to be an effective antimanic agent in older people although there have been no trials in post-stroke mania. It has been reported to be well tolerated by older people and can be safely used in combination with antipsychotics. The recommended starting dose is 125 mg twice a day, gradually increased to reach an optimum dose by monitoring blood levels.
- Carbamazepine is another well-known antimanic agent more widely studied in younger populations. Special attention should be paid to a past history of blood dyscrasias or liver disease as carbamazapine is known to cause bone marrow depression and hepatic toxicity. Starting dose recommended for older people is 200 mg/day and gradually increasing to 400–600 mg/day with monitoring of blood levels.
- Other anticonvulsants like gabapentin and lamotrigine have also been reported to be useful in managing acute mania in the adult population. Their use in post-stroke mania should only be considered as second- or third-line treatments where other treatments have either not worked or cannot be used due to poor tolerability.
- Atypical antipsychotics, such as olanzapine are effective in acute mania. Among older people with dementia, atypical antipsychotics are likely to increase the risk of cerebrovascular accident (CVA).
- Amongst benzodiazepines, lorazepam, a short-acting benzodiazepine, has been shown to be effective in acute mania. It is commonly used as an adjunctive medication for control of behavioural symptoms of mania along with the mood stabilizers that take a longer time to exert their action. The other advantage of lorazepam is its availability in both oral and injectable form, which can be useful in episodes of acute disturbance. The recommended daily dose is 0.5–1 mg oral or IM, which can be repeated up to three to four times in 24 h.

Other post-stroke disorders

Post-stroke anxiety disorder

Post-stroke anxiety disorders are common and present with increased anxiety, excessive fear, worrying, and disturbed sleep.[1] It is important to assess for the possibility of comorbid depression. SSRIs are the first line medical treatment. Benzodiazepines should usually be avoided, and buspirone can be trialled as a second line or adjuvant therapy with antidepressants.

Post-stroke psychosis

- Psychotic illness after stroke should be clearly distinguished from delirium. Sometimes post-stroke depression can present with psychotic features.
- Because of the complexity of diagnostic possibilities and the risk of [illegible] and disorganized behaviour, all patients with post-stroke psychosis should be referred for a psychiatric consultation.
- Atypical antipsychotics are suggested to be the first line of treatment due to their favourable side-effect profile.
- Concerns about the two most commonly used atypical antipsychotics, risperidone and olanzapine, with the possible role in increasing the risk of cerebrovascular disease and stroke, have narrowed the choice of medication. More recent reviews have, however, suggested that the other atypical antipsychotics, including quetiapine and aripiprazole, may share the same risk factors and use of typical antipsychotics may prove more harmful due to their side effects. [illegible] non-demented patients have not been shown to share these risks.
- Patients with a past history of psychotic illness may be treated with the same antipsychotic medication that helped in the past. Conventional antipsychotics are [illegible] with sedative and anticholinergic effects and marked increase in risk of extrapyramidal side effects in the presence of brain disease should be weighed in the decision. Atypicals will usually be favoured and doses lower than those indicated for non-stroke patients may be used initially.
- All new cases should be treated with atypical antipsychotics as first line with the choice of drug depending on the individual patient's situation. Olanzapine with its tendency to increase glucose metabolism should be avoided in diabetic patients. In more elderly patients, quetiapine 25 mg/50 mg titrated up to 400–800 mg/d requires a twice-a-day dose with slow titration and is known to cause sedation and postural hypotension. Modified release quetiapine starting at 50 mg in the elderly and then [illegible] once daily. Risperidone has a higher chance than may [illegible] cause extrapyramidal side effects and may increase the risk of further strokes. Aripiprazole possibly superior side-effect profile and convenient once daily dose might be useful. Post-stroke patients who are likely to be on a number of medications and struggling to recover from their physical disability.

1. [illegible] (2009). [illegible]

Other post-stroke disorders

Post-stroke anxiety disorder

Post-stroke anxiety disorders are common and present with increased anxiety, excessive sweating, worrying, and disturbed sleep.[1] It is important to assess for the possibility of comorbid depression. SSRIs are the first-line medical treatment. Benzodiazepines should usually be avoided and buspirone can be used as a second-line or adjuvant therapy with antidepressants.

Post-stroke psychosis

- A psychotic illness after stroke should be clearly distinguished from delirium. Sometimes post-stroke depression can present with psychotic features.
- Because of the complexity of diagnostic possibilities and the risk of dangerous and disorganized behaviour, all patients with post-stroke psychosis should be referred for a psychiatric consultation.
- Atypical antipsychotics are suggested to be the first line of treatment due to their favourable side-effect profile.
- Concerns about the two most commonly used atypical antipsychotics (risperidone and olanzapine), with their possible role in increasing the risk of cerebrovascular disease and stroke, has narrowed the choice of medication. More recent reviews have, however, suggested that the other atypical antipsychotics, including quetiapine and aripiprazole, may share the same risk factors, and use of typical antipsychotics may prove more harmful due to their side effects. In theory, non-demented patients have not been shown to share these risks.
- Patients with a past history of psychotic illness may be treated with the same antipsychotic medication that helped in the past. Consideration of blood pressure, compliance, sedative and anticholinergic effects, and the marked increase in risk of extrapyramidal side effects in the presence of brain disease should be weighed in the decision. Atypicals will usually be favoured, and doses lower than those initiated in non-stroke patients may be used at first.
- All new cases should be treated with atypical antipsychotics as first line with the choice of drug depending on the individual patient's situation. Olanzapine with its tendency to disturb glucose metabolism should be avoided in diabetic patients. Immediate release quetiapine (e.g. 50 mg BD titrated up to 400–800 mg) requires a twice-a-day dose with slow titration and is known to cause sedation and postural hypertension. Modified release quetiapine starts at 50 mg in the elderly and can be dosed once daily. Risperidone has a higher tendency to cause extrapyramidal side effects and may increase the risk of further strokes. Aripiprazole's possibly superior side-effect profile and convenient once-daily dose might be useful in post-stroke patients who are likely to be on a number of medications and struggling to recover from their physical disabilities.

1 For further information see Bourgeois JA et al. (2005). Post-stroke psychiatric syndromes: diagnosis and pharmacologic intervention. Appl Neurol. Published online 9 February 2005.

References

1. Brzecka A, Leszek J, Ashraf GM, et al. Sleep disorders associated with Alzheimer's disease: A perspective. Front Neurosci. 2018;12:330.
2. Judd BG and Sateia MJ. Classification of sleep disorders. Up To Date 2022. Available from: https://www.uptodate.com/contents/classification-of-sleep-disorders#H618724333
3. Dauvilliers Y, Schenck CH, Postuma RB, et al. REM sleep behaviour disorder. Nat Rev Dis Primers. 2018 2018/08/30;4(1):19.
4. Howell M, Avidan AY, Foldvary-Schaefer N, et al. Management of REM sleep behavior disorder: An American Academy of Sleep Medicine clinical practice guideline. JCSM. 2023;19(4):759–768.
5. Mignot E, Mayleben D, Fietze I, et al. Safety and efficacy of daridorexant in patients with insomnia disorder: Results from two multicentre, randomised, double-blind, placebo-controlled, phase 3 trials. Lancet Neurol. 2022;21(2):125–139.
6. Sateia MJ, Buysse DJ, Krystal AD, et al. Clinical Practice Guideline for the pharmacologic treatment of chronic insomnia in adults: An American Academy of Sleep Medicine Clinical Practice Guideline. JCSM. 2017;13(02):307–349.
7. Santos CO, Caeiro L, Ferro JM, et al. Mania and stroke: a systematic review. Cerebrovasc Dis. 2011;32(1):11–21.

Index

For the benefit of digital users, indexed terms that span two pages (e.g., 52–53) may, on occasion, appear on only one of those pages.

Tables and figures are indicated by an italic *t* and *f* following the page number.

A

D

K

L

M

N

O

W

X

Y

Z